Your Aging Parent

Your Aging Parent

Maxine Dowd Jensen

Published by
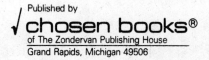
chosen books®
of The Zondervan Publishing House
Grand Rapids, Michigan 49506

Your Aging Parent
Copyright © 1985 by Maxine Dowd Jensen

Chosen Books is an imprint of Zondervan Publishing House,
1415 Lake Drive, S.E., Grand Rapids, Michigan 49506.

Library of Congress Cataloging in Publication Data

Jensen, Maxine Dowd, 1919–
    Your aging parent.

    Includes index.
    1. Family—Religious life.   2. Aged—Religious life.   I. Title.
BV4526.2.J44   1985   646.7'8   85-22800
ISBN 0-310-61071-0

All Scripture quotations, unless otherwise noted, are taken from
the HOLY BIBLE: NEW INTERNATIONAL VERSION (North
American Edition). Copyright © 1973, 1978, 1984, by the
International Bible Society. Used by permission of Zondervan
Bible Publishers.

Edited by Jane Campbell
Designed by Louise Bauer

Printed in the United States of America

85 86 87 88 89 90 91 92 / 8 7 6 5 4 3 2 1

CONTENTS

INTRODUCTION

As I walked toward my desk on the day after New Year's day, I spied a memo pinned on my calendar pad. I had been absent since December 26, the day my mother died.

Detaching the slip, I smiled as I read. Then I laughed. *At my age?* I thought. *With no prospects?* Seeing Vi approach, I shook my finger at her and shoved the paper under her nose. "Take it back. You can't win," I said.

"Oh, but I will."

Once again I glanced at her note.

I.O.U.

If you are not married by one year from today, I will take you to any event and restaurant of your choice.

Vi.

"You did this just to get a laugh out of me. Well, you've succeeded."

Her face became serious. "Yes, I did it for that reason. But my prediction will come true. Your responsibilities have kept you from marriage."

"You're silly. I just never met the right man," I responded.

"Maybe, but I think that subconsciously you didn't want any man to further complicate your life."

Later, mulling over her words, I rejected her reasoning. That was not why I refused to allow my dating to become serious. I remembered a time, however, when I deliberately turned off romance.

I was eighteen and had graduated recently from junior college. Working full-time as a bakery salesgirl, I dreamed of saving my salary and entering Northwestern University in the fall. I planned to become a writer.

Then my dreams dissipated. My father was carried home from work, never to return to his job.

I had been unaware of my father's gradual deterioration. I had noticed that he walked unsteadily. In fact, I was always embarrassed about it, hoping my friends would not think that he was drunk. But I did not recognize the insidious disease that was crippling the control of his arms and his legs.

My mother, however, had realized what was happening and had walked him to a busy street each morning. She had watched as he crossed and headed for the railroad yards. Each afternoon she had sat in the window awaiting his return.

When he was brought home, the few dollars he had managed to tuck away as the Depression waned soon disappeared. The doctors we sought out could not reverse the progress of his disease.

During this period, Al and I met. Perhaps the times we spent together made me happy because I hesitated to face my future, a future I realized included the financial care of my parents. My young father possessed too few years of service for a pension; his company had no disability program. My mother ran the household, and my father would need her at home. In those days—not long ago—social security was new, and state disability insurance was not yet mandated by law.

But that year as Christmas drew near, I forced myself to consider the future. I knew Al planned to slip an engagement ring onto my finger just as surely as I knew his sights were set on the ministry. At that time, churches did not allow the minister's wife to work; they expected two employees for the price of one. His starting salary would never support four adults. What if we had children? I found it difficult to envision terminating our relationship.

Even in the days after I said good-by, however,

when I refused to take Al's calls and replied to my mother's troubled questions with, "It wasn't meant to be," I felt the undergirding of my God. I believe He directed my decision. Didn't He say, "Honor thy father and mother"?

As I look back, I *know* that decision was right. I was too young and not yet ready to be a wife. My all-seeing God glimpsed the six days of regular work plus ten hours extra every Sunday that would be required of me.

I like to believe God wanted my marriage to epitomize what He created a marriage to be. He knew that, at eighteen, I was not prepared.

I finally admitted all this to myself as I thought again about Vi's words. If I had not cared for Al, I might have dumped my responsibilities onto his shoulders, sought the shelter of his arms, and let him wrestle with the knots in my life.

Could Vi be right? I wondered. *Had my personal problems been a subconscious reason for running the other way when an eligible man started serious pursuit?*

In the years between my decision about Al and the deaths of my father and mother, I discovered that romance is only one of the problems adult children face when parents become dependent in some way or when one parent loses the other because of divorce or death.

I also learned that our all-caring Father God knows our personal dreams. Over the years, He has slowly brought me the fulfillment of mine. He can do the same for you.

My hair is now salted with silver, and someday soon I may join the ranks of the approximately 27 million aging Americans who either need forms of assistance or are approaching this period. Some will be valiant and self-sufficient to the end. Others may worry about their financial future, where they will live, their physical well-being, and how their children will react when age forces a physical or mental slowdown.

Adult children struggle almost unaided with the problems of their aging parents. Doctors and nurses often find it difficult to minister to the aged. These professionals admit that medical and nursing schools give little attention to the study of the elderly.

Adult children care about their parents. Because of the lack of resource material, however, they often push the anticipated problem aside, experience guilt feelings, or worry about how the dependency of a parent will affect their personal life.

If you are such a child, this book has been written to help you learn to cope. My prayer is that it will lift your spirits, show you practical solutions, and enable you to face the future with a confident, victorious attitude.

I have weathered over twenty years of living with, loving, and supporting an ill father, a dependent mother, and a stroke victim mother-in-law. I've learned that nothing is as bad as it looks. All problems are solvable. Personal goals can be realized. Romance before or after marriage can be retained. Individuality, peace, and love are available for all the persons involved.

While looking after my parents, I observed friends struggling with similar and different situations. These friends, in addition to some doctors and ministers, cooperated as I prepared this book. I sought solutions based on different types of personalities and problems. They responded.

Many of the difficulties you face are common. Only people vary, as do their solutions and reactions.

This book will show you ways of coping or of obtaining help. The future you face need not fill you with dread. The coming years can be blessed ones. They can be filled with loving and caring and mutual respect as you work for happiness and individuality. There is a way out, around, or through any problems you face.

Dr. Bertram B. Moss, in his book *Caring for the Aged,* says, "Don't despair when faced with a 'problem parent.' There may be an answer to your parent's problem."

God says, "My grace is sufficient for you . . ." (2 Corinthians 12:9a).

The end result of honoring our parents—the only commandment with a promise (Exodus 20:12)—will be peace of mind and a host of fond memories.

1
Where Are You Now?

The ringing telephone pierced my dream. I looked at the clock, then at my husband groping for the receiver. It was 5:35 A.M. I began to bury my head in the pillow, but the sudden sharpness of his voice startled me. My eyes flew open. Sleep fled.

We rose, slipped into our clothes and headed for the hospital. When we arrived, my mother-in-law smiled from one side of her mouth and tried to speak.

Though her stroke shocked us, we were not unprepared. My husband and I had discussed the future possibility of her need to live with us. We had added a dormer and a complete bath on the second floor of our bungalow, just in case.

On the long ride to the hospital, however, I thought, *Will I have to quit work? Can I handle a stroke victim?*

I never had to answer. My mother-in-law bounced back. She moved in with us. Then another stroke hit her, and she died before the end of the following month.

The Bible tells us our life is "a mist that appears for a little while and then vanishes" (James 4:14). We don't know how long we, or those we love, will live. Will good health continue?

Maybe you are saying, "I don't want to think about these things." If so, you are normal. Most of us do not want to face the fact that our parents, who have always been there *for* us, may someday depend *on* us. Consider this because our greatest problem, at the beginning, is with ourselves.

We may hope our parents will remain healthy and

on their own. We may even avoid visiting them because we think they may ask us about their future. Instead of this, consider what your reactions would have been if you had awakened to a similar early morning call. What questions would have flooded your mind?

Be honest. Would you have been resentful? Worried? Afraid?

Resentment can take various forms. "Why is this happening right now?" "Will I have to change jobs because I travel?" "How can I take care of Dad? I need all the extra room." "Harry's so close to retirement. The kids are on their own. There goes our second honeymoon." "I'm not well. I have all I can do to take care of my husband and myself." "I love Mom/Dad, but I'll be stuck."

Such resentment will dissipate if you remember that it is not wrong to want to keep some distance between your life and that of your parents. Nor should you despair if you desire freedom to pursue a career or a dream. But it is dreadfully wrong not to show consideration. This is one of the things we owe our parents.

We also owe them respect. This may prove difficult for some people. If so, substitute understanding and compassion.

We owe loyalty. According to Webster, loyalty is faithful devotion, and devotion often leads to worry. If you must worry, and some of us are built that way, try to do it positively.

Willis H. Carrier, the engineer who launched the air-conditioning industry, had a recipe for this problem. He analyzed the situation, figured out the worst possible result, and determined to accept this result, if necessary. Then he began working to avoid the worst.

Try these principles while admitting the possibility that someday your parents will not be totally independent. Submit to this truth and adjust.

Submitting and adjusting are not all bad. What some people call a "cross," others do not consider a burden at all. If you rebel, you become bitter and miserable. If you adjust, the low moments can be fleeting ones.

Accept the vulnerability of your parents. Promise yourself that you will do your best if the worst happens. Then relax.

Lin Yutang, philosopher and author, believed that releasing the mind from worry was to energize it for working out solutions. Since one of your main worries may center on what other people must think, remember that Shakespeare said, ". . . to thine own self be true. . . ." Don't make yourself unhappy by fretting about the opinions of others. If you are true to yourself, people around you will sense your serenity. Everything will be easier.

Dr. Manuel J. Smith, in his book *When I Say No I Feel Guilty,* says, "You have the right to offer no reasons or excuses to justify your behavior." Some parents have a difficult time accepting this. They expect us to explain ourselves or do exactly what they ask.

My mother-in-law sometimes complained because my husband smoked. She overlooked the facts that he controlled his smoking, that his hands had never acquired a nicotine stain, that he was considerate of others, and that he never exuded a stale tobacco smell. When my husband and I were alone, he would mutter, "I'm a grown man with adult children. Why does she still treat me like a naughty little boy?"

Your behavior and beliefs may evoke not only worry but also fear of arguments. Will you make excuses and try to justify yourself?

There is a better way. Try listening to the other person; then request the same courtesy. Speak in an even voice. This will calm rather than ignite feelings. Agree to consider the other person's point of view.

Later, discuss the matter further, or do as I did when my sister-in-law felt I had my glasses, dishes, and silverware in all the wrong places. I listened. I said, "Maybe you're right." Then I changed not even one teaspoon.

Don't fear an argument. Keep your conversation as light, as full of humor, and as equipped with tolerance as possible. Most of the arguments, feelings, doubts, and worries you dread can be resolved. Your attitude can determine many of the results. Remember, it is not what happens to you that spoils life but how you react to what happens.

Learn to pray this prayer:

O God, give us serenity to accept what cannot be changed, courage to change what should be changed, and wisdom to distinguish the one from the other.

Dr. Reinhold Niebuhr

Stop. Think. Then dare to act. Never succumb to the view that there is no way out and no answer. Above all else, remember we can do all things through Christ who strengthens us.

2
Preplanning for Camelot

One of the things we must not fear is consideration of the future of our aging parents.

"When is the best time to discuss these later years with my parents?" a friend asked. "I can't barge in and say, 'You're getting old, Ma, Pa. Shouldn't you think about your future?'"

As your parents grow older, think through possible alternatives for their future. When the appropriate time arrives, you can furnish educated suggestions. These will show your parents your interest, your concern, and your love.

Think first about leaving your parents right where they are. Ann Landers and many others have said, "The ideal solution is to keep the surviving parent (or parents) in his or her own home." This need not be the house in which they now live. It may be an apartment or place in a retirement community, a mobile home, or a condominium. The grounds should be small and easily cared for or kept up by the management.

If you believe in God, pray about this.

Someday, after your parents have mentioned possible retirement, broach the subject of where they plan to live. Let them know you are not nosy; you care about their future and have given it thought. Most parents will appreciate your willingness to listen to their ideas *before* any emergency arises.

Of course, your parents, like you, may not want to face the realities of the future. If they do not, try the drip-drop method. I often used this when I wished to soften up my parents. Plant an idea here and a thought there. Later, you may find them considering your suggestions.

Today many older people can count on a company pension, social security, bank accounts, or financial investments. Many elderly people own their own homes.

If your parents are financially able to continue living in their present location, they may be happiest there. The things around them—family, friends, stores, community activities, their church—will all be familiar.

If your parents bought their house when you and your siblings lived there, however, the home may be too large, and the yard may require too much work. Or their house may have several levels, making it difficult for them to get around. Unless the living room, dining area, kitchen, and at least one bedroom and one bath are all on one floor, it may be wiser and safer for your parents to move. Discuss this with them. See what their feelings are.

You may discover they wish to retire to a senior citizens' community in a vacation area. If so, inquire about the pitfalls as well as the blessings of living in this kind of community.

Is the place they desire far from you? If so, what transportation is available?

No matter where they live, if your mother does not know how to drive, encourage her to learn. If your father dies and your mother knows how to drive, she can live in any place that seems like home instead of being forced to relocate. Remind her that knowing how to drive can also help in some emergency situations. Her ability to drive might even prove lifesaving on a vacation trip. Some men feel the twinges of a heart attack but keep on driving because their wives cannot drive.

My community in Arkansas is nearly ideal—except for transportation. The nearest large airport is 125 miles away. The community has no train service; it offers only a commuter-type bus that goes to the town with the airport or to another town, a distance of 160 miles. The hours of this bus do not always coincide with air time, and an overnight stay in a motel, plus meals, are added expenses. A seven-passenger shuttle plane does fly to another large city, but this adds an extra $125 or $150 to the cost of the trip. Recently, the only taxi in town went out of business.

Urge your parents to investigate the transportation alternatives in their proposed Eden. Some condominiums and retirement villages supply a bus. Some areas have senior citizens' pickup services. Neighbors in friendly sections often share rides.

Is transportation available in case of illness? Are there volunteer services or is there a hospice in the area? My area has a hospice that does not limit its care to the terminally ill. As a volunteer, I have taken semi-incapacitated people to the store, to the beauty shop, and to distant hospitals.

Remind your parents that they must take future illness into consideration when they move away. How adequate are the nearby medical facilities? What types of doctors are located there?

If one of them becomes ill and the other does not drive, they may be forced to rely on a new friend for transportation. Will either of them be too proud to accept help on a long-term basis? If one of them must go to a distant hospital, will they be able to afford the cost of an ambulance or plane as well as food and lodging for the spouse who waits while the ill spouse is being treated? It can be this or separation.

Every day in my community, people travel to Houston, Texas or Springfield, Missouri or Little Rock, Arkansas to obtain medical treatment. A long ambulance or airplane ride can contribute to the death or additional disability of a patient, since in some instances speed of treatment is one of the greatest factors in saving a life or preventing serious aftereffects. Such aftereffects or even symptoms of an undiscovered illness can remove the joy from retirement.

Explain that you want your parents to live for today, but ask them to consider the long-range possibilities of what they will do if they cannot take care of themselves.

Right now I know of several widows and at least three couples who desperately need to sell their homes and move to an area with better transportation and medical care. They face additional problems if they cannot sell their houses for the appraised value. They may seriously jeopardize their future finances.

In the selection of a new location, your parents should consider recreational and educational facilities. Encourage them to subscribe to the local paper. They can discover many facets of the prospective community. Check this paper for hobbies they intend to pursue. Would your mother like a part-time or full-time job? Look at the help wanted columns. Will your father make your mother a golf or fishing widow? Will she forsake him for card parties? Will one of your parents resist the efforts of the other to follow some regular or proposed new interest? Will the other parent become frustrated?

Because one woman's husband scoffs at her dreams of becoming a writer, she is writing at 5:00 A.M. while he sleeps. A similar situation could happen if your parents remain in their original location, although old friends would be close at hand and stores, parks, and recreational activities would be familiar.

Recreation is seldom a problem in a mobile-home park. Shuffleboard courts, tennis courts, swimming pools, and clubhouses abound. This is also true of many condominium complexes that may feature planned activities, such as card parties, square-dance lessons, Saturday morning coffees, Bible studies, bike hikes (three-wheelers acceptable), as well as cruises and trips to faraway places or to some nearby dinner theater or historical area.

This may not be true if your parents buy a home. Some neighbors resent a "snow-bird" living on their street. A part-time job agency may tell the well-qualified secretary, "We didn't call you before but now we're scraping the bottom of the barrel." (This actually happened to my sister-in-law.)

Will your parents fit in if they move south of the Mason-Dixon line, if they are Yankees in Rebel territory? Will they understand the local phrases and translate the accent?

Your parents should consider whether they make friends easily. Do relatives or long-time friends already live in the area they have chosen? Will old friends be able or willing to travel that far?

What about the weather? Arizona is unbeatable during the winter and spring, but it can be stifling and unbearable in the summer. Will your parents have financial resources to leave during unpleasant times? Or will they do as the sister of a friend of mine who barricades herself in her home in summer? She is afraid among the vacant houses.

Florida can be a paradise, but love-bugs appear every six months. Sometimes the bugs are so thick that drivers have to stop to clean their windshields.

Will the humidity that drips each morning from a porch overhang prove to be a constant irritation? Will your mother appreciate guarding clothing from mildew and guarding flour and crackers from weevils or flying cockroaches?

A friend of mine who has lived in Miami since age nineteen still shudders during hurricane season. A hurricane is surpassed in ferocity only by the tornado.

Suggest that your parents visit their proposed Utopia in its worst season. If they like it then, they will love it as its best.

How about shopping? Will they have to travel 125 miles to buy a good electric blanket or a fluorescent bulb to fit the bathroom fixture? If items are ordered, will it take ten days to receive the gift certificate of a national catalog house? When they get the product, will they find they have paid a dollar more than the one friends brought when visiting?

Will your parents expect you and the grandchildren to visit on *every* vacation? It may prove a lark if a boat is at your disposal for fishing and water-skiing, or it could be a drag. Will your mother pine for the grandchildren? Will this cause friction?

Discuss this aspect. You should want to see them often, but their suggested place may allow little choice.

Think, too, of things that please your parents. If music or art is an integral part of their life, what will be the opportunities for its pursuit? Will they feel stifled because each turn of the dial means rock and roll or country music, since no educational channel is available? Will they find it necessary to spend weekends in a distant city in order to attend a classical concert or well-acted play? They may even have to travel far to buy records. The local store may never seem to receive what is ordered.

Keep your parents from making mistakes. You can go far in that direction if you will preplan with them.

What does your mother think of your father's retirement? She may be a fast disappearing breed, having remained at home because of moral convictions or financial freedom. Now that retirement approaches for your father, is she looking forward to it? She may dread it, imagining it will curtail her liberty.

You can help her. Explain that both she and your father deserve leisure time apart and together. Encourage her to find new activities they can share while not giving up all of her present ones. Channel her toward the second honeymoon idea. You know them both. Pray for wisdom and assist them.

As you plan the things you will discuss, you should be aware of some attendant problems. Are your parents financially secure and able to pay for the services they will need? If not, how will they manage? You might want to check the widows' rights in the state where they will retire. Some of these still consider a woman a chattel with no more rights of inheritance than if she were a chair her husband sat on.

Do you have sisters or brothers? Will they cooperate financially or personally?

Does your parent have a trait or habit that annoys you? Have you learned to cope with it?

How much time should you share with your parents? Find a happy medium between smothering and neglect.

Do you know when to say yes to your parents? Should you ever say no?

In your childhood you were expected to obey your parents' rules. What precepts should be followed now, and who should compose them?

Do you have a dream, a goal, an objective for your life? Is there a chance that, with the retirement of your parents, it will be scuttled? Should you abandon it, wait for it, or, damning the torpedoes, go after it?

Of course, you don't have to make all these decisions now. You can wait for each incident to arise. Planning ahead, however, is never wrong. Plans can be scrapped.

Remember, too, that independence and "selfishness" are not all bad. You have a right to keep your home life apart. Just don't forget to provide love and warmth and an independent place for your parents.

You might be interested to know that Singapore's Prime Minister, Lee Kuan Yew, is worried about the tendency of the young to fail to consider their parents. In his Chinese New Year Message for 1982 he said, "We must reverse the trend for all married children to

... leave their parents to live by themselves." He believes Asian societies have survived without state welfare systems because of their tradition of venerating elders.

If children of aging parents will, in love, provide proper homes for their own, all ages will be happier and the economy of our nation helped. These residences do not need to be a combination of generations to accomplish loving care. In fact, the best possible way, in our country, is for each family to be independent. It is possible for you to arrange this.

3
Providing That Independent Place

How can you help your parents continue to be independent? Look around. Many people, even into their eighties and nineties, are self-sufficient. Allow your parent to be free to choose as long as possible.

One loving son failed to do this. His widowed mother settled into a creative, productive life while he served in the Navy. Afterward, while attending an out-of-state college, he insisted she move to the same town. He graduated and accepted a job in another state. She begged to return to her original home, but he tried to show his love by wanting her nearby. Understanding his wishes, she surrendered. When the son teetered on the edge of a nervous breakdown, however, his doctor said, "You must not live with your mother."

The son sought out a fine nursing home since his mother had a slight heart condition. She lived in that home for fourteen years. She died when she was eighty-six. How much better it would have been if the mother had remained in her former home!

Listen to your parent. Hear what he or she is saying. Listen not only with your mind but also with your heart.

Of course, your parent may stand up to you. Another son tried to convince his seventy-eight-year-old mother, victim of a broken arm, to enter a retirement home with hospital facilities. He, too, cared. He did not learn of her accident, however, until after she set off on a trip to New Zealand and Australia. (Had she kept it from him because she knew he would have discouraged her?) "Listen," she said. "If I can figure out which clothes to carry, wash, and put on while away; if I can manage to eat and sign checks left-handed, I can manage my own home. And if I can't, a woman who can afford such a trip can pay for household help!"

Let your parents express their opinions. They may be right. After all, they have weathered many storms in the past.

Financial ability, however, may dictate their future circumstances. My mother-in-law needed my husband's help in budgeting her finances when the people buying the old family home on contract suddenly obtained a mortgage and paid off the balance.

Perhaps you can do as my husband did. Since his mother allowed him access to her records, he set up a budget for her. He cautioned her on only one thing—her philanthropy.

She fretted. She hated to cut back her giving to God. I settled it amicably by saying, "You've given over and above your tithe for many years. God must keep records. He knows you've paid far in advance." This tickled her. She accepted her new budget.

If you are allowed to assist your parent, you may discover his or her eligibility for a pension. You may find that a realignment of assets will garner more income.

Be prepared, though, to find out some things you would rather not know. Your parent may have been subsidizing your sibling or some grandchild while giving only token gifts to you and yours. If so, still your tongue. Your parent has this right, fair or not.

You may find that funds are inadequate to maintain the house in which your parents live. If so, discuss a smaller place.

Some elderly people refuse to move. They are attached to memories or keepsakes. If so, try to discover what things they treasure. Keep these in mind and measure them. Then see where the items could fit in a new location.

Check apartment buildings and hotels in your town. Some may be turning into private quarters for the elderly. The apartments may be tiny but comfortable.

A gentleman I know in Abilene, Kansas, enjoys a hot meal delivered every day, a weekly housecleaning, and close proximity to stores, churches, and entertainment. Neighbors keep tabs on each other.

When you take your parents to view these spots, explain where the comfortable rocker could stand, where the satin-smooth mahogany buffet might sit, where a favorite picture could be hung.

If you show respect for your parents' wishes, you may be surprised by their cooperation. A smile is contagious and so is an understanding heart.

Some parents, however, may grow more stubborn and balk at change. If so, enlist the help of a doctor, social service worker, minister, priest, or rabbi. You may need the personal contact of one of their friends.

Most parents wish to remain independent. Let them know that you, too, want them to control their own life.

But what if your parent wishes to remain independent, is having financial problems, and refuses to accept monetary help? Surely you can think up a solution.

One of my friends worked out this problem in the following way. She remembered that her father and his deceased brother had purchased property in a distant state. One day she wrote her cousin. "If I send money earmarked for my dad, will you make up an excuse for those properties to pay off, then forward the money to him?" It worked. Her father delighted in these unexpected "windfalls."

Also consider the services necessary if your parents are to remain independent. You can contact a senior citizens' agency or a social service agency. These can point you in the right direction.

If your parent is not physically able to clean the house, do the repairs, and care for the yard, you have two options: Do the work yourself or select a competent worker. If your parent is afraid of strangers in the home, you may decide to enlist the aid of your brothers and sisters. One daughter I know fixes broken stairsteps, cleans the windows and gutters, does heavy household duties and numerous other tasks for her mother. A son mows the lawn.

When you plan to do these things, avoid friction in your own home as well as theirs by setting a definite time when you are available. We all know emergencies arise. Washing machines flood the floors, fuses blow, a baseball can crash through a window. But only an emergency should intrude on your personal time.

Once you have made arrangements for various services, you may discover that stopping in or calling every day is neither necessary nor desired. Many areas offer a telephone service that will phone your parent at a specific time every day. Or neighbors and friends keep in touch. When such arrangements are used, be sure your telephone number is known. This will ensure that you are informed, if needed.

Even if there is some daily provision, don't stop your own calls. Show interest. If your parents become bored, have some ideas on tap.

One of these many involve gardening. Have they shown interest in gardening but have not had an opportunity? If they live in an apartment, they can grow strawberries in hanging baskets, parsley in a windowbox, and tomatoes or other vegetables in a pot on their balcony. Orchids, African violets, and cacti also can be interesting to raise.

What about people-oriented ideas? Kitchen bands and choral groups often meet in the daytime. Various areas have quilting bees and sewing circles. People involved in these activities often bring a sack lunch. Your mother could even instigate such an activity.

A number of men in our town have become woodcarvers. They travel to competitions, win prizes, display, and sell their wares.

These things all help, but the most important factor that keeps your parents independent is the way they eat.

An aunt of mine lives across the street from a park where hot meals are served on weekdays. After the meal card tables are set up. Frisky oldsters challenge each other at ping-pong; eagle-eyed men and women knock balls into billiard-table pockets; and several people gather around an upright piano where someone exercises arthritic fingers while others sing lustily.

The Meals on Wheels organization is active in many communities. Assure your parents that this is not charity. Churches serve meals. The cost is stated by a member of the committee or the price is printed on an envelope. They are free to give more or less. If your parents don't want to be delivered to, they may wish to deliver. Serving gets people away from their four walls, talking to each other and feeling useful. Eating out gets your parents into fresh air, allows them to be with people, and is easier than fixing a meal at home.

Mealtime can be an unhappy period. One woman I have heard about buys day-old pastries, and whenever she is hungry, she takes one out of the refrigerator and eats it. Some elderly people have cereal for dinner. It isn't much work. But on such a diet, malnutrition, ill health, and even death can result.

Some women simply grow tired of cooking. Can you make it fun for them? You can try.

Speed in preparation helps. Microwave ovens are fast. Give your mother a gift of one or suggest she buy it.

For instance, your parent can roast meat in the conventional oven, then cut and freeze it. Sliced roast, placed in a microwave oven along with leftover mashed potatoes and an accompanying vegetable, can taste like freshly cooked food in thirty seconds. This makes a pot roast or rolled roast economical.

One recently widowed friend, who is eighty years old, bought herself a microwave. Last Saturday she attended a class on how to use it. Another woman has tried every recipe in the cookbook that was included at the time of purchase. Encourage your parents to learn to use one.

Another speedy approach to cooking might work for your parents. A raw egg beaten up in orange juice makes a tasty, nutritious breakfast.

A cooking binge works, too. Several pounds of ground beef, some stew meat, two or three chicken breasts, and four or five pork chops can be purchased and cooked at the same time. Bake the chicken and pork; simmer the stew and prepare small meatloaves; prepare a ground beef mixture by adding onions, green pepper, and canned tomatoes to the browned meat. Use the ground beef mixture as a base for sloppy joes and chili, or serve it over rice or noodles. When the food is cooked, it can be wrapped separately or put into small containers and frozen. This method is the fastest way I know to have a nutritious meal without a microwave. When the main part of the meal needs only to be heated, your parent will be more likely to throw a handful of frozen vegetables into a pot, prepare a salad, and have a good meal.

Occasionally prepare a tasty dish and take part of it to your parent for freezing and future eating.

An elderly widow friend received a meal-in-a-bag appliance from her children. It turns out a prepared meal that is easy to heat up and has her own flavorings.

My youngest daughter gave me a three-divisional Nordic skillet one year. You can also buy similar T-fal ones. With these, previously cooked meat can be warmed up, cups of vegetables added from the large freezer bags, or insipid-tasting apples sliced and flavored with butter, cinnamon, and brown sugar; and all can be cooked at once.

Suggest that your parent ask the butcher to cut a pot roast or rump roast into several pieces. Freeze them uncooked. These provide an excuse to invite someone to join the evening meal.

A greatly admired friend of mine pampers herself. She prepares a good, hot meal every day. If she doesn't want to miss a TV show, she arranges her meal on a snack table. If the day is beautiful, she eats at a tiny table on her balcony. Often she buys a flower or two and puts the vase on her dinner table. Mealtime is a luxurious treat that she squanders on herself alone.

Another friend has raised a family and is now retired. She says the only way she can keep cooking is to try new recipes. Her husband is willing to eat anything, and her children often drop in for a meal.

Also try to interest your parents in other new things. Your mother can enter a cooking contest or send the details of her best dishes to a home magazine. Your father may hanker to putter in the kitchen. Winning a prize or receiving a check may revitalize their interest.

There is still another way to whet your parents' appetites. Give gifts of food. These may be welcome if you choose wisely.

Is your father a Scandinavian? What about some herring? (Do not bring caramels, however, if your parent wears dentures!)

There are fruit and meat clubs. Buy a year's gift and your parent will receive something different every month.

If you live close to your parents, invite them often for dinner. Vary the day. That keeps the invitation interesting and at the same time gives you more freedom in case a delightful outing presents itself. You wouldn't want to hurt your parents by canceling an invitation.

When your mother and father visit, prepare additional food. Send the surplus home with them.

In a final effort to help your parents eat nutritiously, stoop to snoop. Raid the icebox, cupboards, and cookie jar as you did when you were a kid. It will increase your knowledge of what your parent is or is not eating.

If your parents look unhealthy or if you are worried about them, do not hesitate to examine the garbage can. One woman whose garbage was picked up every two weeks insisted she was eating. When her daughter lifted the lids of the garbage cans, she found nothing. There should be bags, boxes, cans, even bottles.

The above are all tips to help your parents remain healthy, happy, and independent as long as they desire it. You will think of other methods because you know your parents. If you should run out of ideas, ask God for wisdom. James 1:5 promises that He will give it willingly.

4
Another Independent Way

At one time in my subdivision, six houses were occupied by widows. Why didn't we join forces? Probably because we were all so different.

Tolerance is a cornerstone for a sharing arrangement. A division of tasks is also necessary.

In one instance I know about, the first woman is a fabulous cook but hates housework. The second dislikes cooking but loves to tear into all the corners. The first woman is frightened of climbing a ladder, so the other cleans gutters, changes light bulbs, and paints ceilings. Household tasks can be shared if your parent decides to join forces with another person. Suggest, however, that they agree on a few rules. This is best because personality traits and likes and dislikes can be deterrents to the "sharing-a-home" concept.

Nevertheless, combining households should be considered as a way for a parent to remain independent. It is economical, it will reinforce security, and it can be satisfying.

The best union is probably between siblings or other relatives. In Denver, a brother lived alone until his sister's husband died. Now the brother and sister share her mobile home. They travel individually with friends or to their children. Their home is never unoccupied.

Two widowed sisters in a Chicago suburb sold their individual homes. Not wanting to live with their children, they bought a condominium together. They both like to entertain and invite many friends into their new place. These women have an understanding that if house guests are primarily the friends of only one of them, she is the one who plans the meals and does most of the cooking, even if she is the housekeeping partner.

The same kind of arrangement can apply to material possessions. Many people fear they will lose prized treasures or disagree over who gets what if they separate. Solve this problem by marking personal items. Appliances and other large goods can be marked with the identification tools that can be borrowed from many local police stations.

Contents of a linen closet as well as keepsakes in a breakfront can be divided. One person can take the left side; the other can take the right.

Prior to moving in together, the people will want to discuss and divide up the living expenses. These can be renegotiated if needs and usage change.

Before the moving in takes place, decide that no piece of furniture will be bought or replaced by splitting the cost. Following this pattern means each is free to move at any time, for any reason, without the hassle of who wants what.

The sharing of a home arrangement by two people who are not related is much more logical today than in the past when daughters or sons remained at home. There is more asserting of independence today, and you, the child, may possess a wise selfishness that says, "I want to do my own thing in my own place."

Because this is so, encourage a lone parent to consider the sharing arrangement. It might mean selling two homes and buying one that allows separate bedrooms and baths while combining recreation rooms, kitchens, and entertaining areas. It can be worth it.

This concept is happening on a larger scale in parts of Florida. Shared homes for five or more people are available. These do away with the institutionalized feeling.

When a larger number of people live together, ample differences of thought stimulate discussions.

There will always be "two or three ... gathered together in my name. . ." (Matthew 18:20 KJV). A fourth partner for bridge is available, as well as someone with whom to shop, to browse in the library, or to explore a park or museum.

Check out the sharing arrangement for your parent. It can provide another independent way.

5
Joining the Generations

After you have thought of all other ways to keep your parents independent, consider joining forces. Will it work? It can.

Dr. Maurice E. Linden, a specialist and former director of Philadelphia's Division of Mental Health, said, "Most children make their elderly parents feel loved and wanted. . . . This is what parents need."

Love your parent. Then remember that the Bible asks, "Do two walk together unless they have agreed to do so?" (Amos 3:3). *Before* you double up, think about and discuss the things that are most important to you.

Just as money and its use can wreck a marriage, so it can cause a major upheaval in the merger of two generations. The actual division of expenses does matter.

The first thing to consider is the ability to pay.

A male friend of mine, an only child, has three children in college, one in high school, one in junior high, and he has just started a business. If his parents become unable to stay in their house, his house will provide adequate space, but for several years ahead he may not be able to shoulder any added expense. My oldest stepdaughter will soon have three sons in college. Her husband is seeking a job following retirement from the Air Force. Neither of these families can bear the additional cost of a parent.

But what if these older folks are living on a fixed income, paying high insurance rates, or catching up on exorbitant medical bills? Some who need to join households may be too young for social security.

You will always have bills to pay—the lights, the

gas, the water, the garbage pickup. These may show little increase with the addition of another person, but you need financial facts.

One son and family moved in with this son's mother. They thought they had settled the problem of who pays what, but they didn't have all the facts. Because of a particular state law, the taxes of this widow were always refunded. Her son was unable to convince her of this. He ended up paying half of them in order to keep peace in the family.

Will peace reign when the monthly bills arrive? Should you divide the costs evenly? If not, how much is equitable? Should it be a static amount or should it fluctuate?

The answers to these questions may depend on how many are in each family and what use they make of the facilities. However, these are important considerations. Decide *beforehand.*

You will need to make other financial decisions. Will the person joining the household pay board and room? Will brothers and sisters contribute?

If you watch a sibling show no care for the welfare of your parent, look out for bitterness in yourself. Remember the ounce of prevention adage, and don't hesitate to discuss the matter.

When figuring up the approximate cost, include everything plus clothing and day-to-day necessities. Place your figures before your parents first, then your brothers and sisters. Ask what each will be able to contribute.

If disputes arise, remain as calm as possible. God's Word tells us, *"If it is possible, . . .* live at peace with everyone" (Romans 12:18, italics added).

Peace was absent in the home of a friend who perhaps did not preplan. The parents of this friend moved in after her father became bedridden. These parents had a good monthly income and offered to pay.

I do not know how the monthly sum was determined, but my friend was never happy about it. One possible solution would have been to renegotiate.

You can do this. Present facts: the dollars-and-cents bottom line. Ask, "What do you think we should do?" Suggest a solution. The division of responsibility should not be ironclad but flexible.

Supporting a parent is a time for bearing one another's burdens—not just the cares of your parents but the needs of other family members as well. A brother who has three children in college should be allowed to cut back on his support. A sister whose children are gone may pick up the difference. A house may burn down; a husband may become incapacitated. That relative needs support, not a drain on finances.

Like Rachel, Jacob, and Esau, some families do not work together. The oldest child in a family I knew remained with her parent. Through the years, living 400 miles from a sister and brother, she supported this mother. My friend's sister occasionally gave money, but the friend's childless brother bought his mother one winter coat and felt he had done his duty. When the mother stopped thinking straight, more home duties fell upon my friend. Then it became too dangerous to leave the mother alone. This tied the daughter to the home. When her mother became incontinent, my friend tried to get her brother to pay for diaper service and a cleaning lady once a week. He refused. Finally, several months before the mother died at age ninety, he sent a pittance.

This situation sounds unforgivable, yet it happens all the time. If it is occurring in your life, do something about it, *now*.

When dividing financial responsibilities, be sure you know what the law says about the support you give. With the 1981 changes in the law, Sylvia Porter suggests in her syndicated newspaper column that you make sure you meet the more-than-half support test and protect your dependency deductions. Ms. Porter advises watching this test closely to make sure you continue to meet it.

In the same column she said that if you are responsible for both parents, you can allocate your support solely to the one who has less income. Your mother's bills may be made out to her but pay these with your check. Keep the bills and canceled checks as your proof and pay all year-end bills promptly.

If your parents provide some childcare for you by babysitting, check the yearly tax books. They will inform you how to report and obtain deductible credits for this.

We have been discussing foreseeable financial problems, but sometimes a financial problem will strike suddenly. What will you do if you are fired or laid off? Do you have a nest egg? I didn't. Nor was I able to accumulate any assets after my father's death. However, God, as He promised, supplied all my need.

After my mother's last operation and while she was still in the hospital, she asked me, "How are you doing for money?"

I laughed and said, "Oh, I keep putting it out, but God seems to keep supplying it."

My parent-child relationship had been a turnabout situation since I turned eighteen. After my father's forecasted death three years later, I gave my mother a small allowance. I gave it to her only when I had a surplus after paying the bills.

I remember the light in her eyes when she later presented me with $100 to help pay for a new living room rug. I remember how she lovingly picked out a Christmas pin for a peer and a doll for a favorite child.

The day she asked me the money question, she told me about a bag sewn into one of her old full-length girdles. Had she died on the operating table before asking, I would have thrown out that dilapidated thing—secret and all. It may pay you, therefore, to give your parent some pocket money. Like bread cast upon waters, it can return when you need it most.

Of course, your income may dictate what you do about living arrangements. Don't feel guilty about your decision if you work it out in love. Perhaps your health or the health of a member of your immediate family will dictate your choice.

I suffered from hay fever. I told my mother that unless I found help for my allergy, I intended to move to the Pacific Northwest. I found an allergist, however, who helped me. I stayed put. Both my mother and I were happy.

Your medical condition may necessitate a move. Should you tell your parent, "This is how it has to be"? Certainly you should if health and happiness rest on that decision.

Even Jesus, while hanging on the cross, remembered His mother. He cared. The Scripture says that from that hour the disciple took her to his own home. Jesus knew this was the best solution for her. Your solution may rest on the advantages and disadvantages of three alternatives: moving in with your parents, moving them in with you, or purchasing an entirely new home.

You may find financial advantage in pooling the money from the sale of both houses. If so, be careful to select a practical home. You will want to purchase one that has a good resale value.

If you build a house in an area where rental apartments are allowed, your problem will evaporate. Build a house that includes a small, separate apartment with its own private entrance.

If zoning does not allow two-family dwellings, however, build an extra bedroom, bath, and sitting room in which concealed cooking facilities are possible.

So many practical electrical appliances are available today that your parents can cook without having a kitchen. Place your utility room adjacent to their cooking area and set up a sink that will serve for soaking clothes or washing dishes.

If you decide to sell one house and remodel the other, you may need the best remodeling person possible. The carpenter can suggest where a house can be expanded, redone, or rearranged. As you make these changes, check for resale value features.

If you propose to use a basement, be sure it is dry. Many older people develop arthritis and allergies to mold. A damp area would not be wise.

A builder may recommend a guest house. This would eliminate difficulties of another kind—those of personality conflicts and annoying habits. If you share the same roof, however, level these to a minimum.

Ask yourself the following questions:

What changes have occurred in my parents' lifestyle and my lifestyle? Will these mesh?

Will we have personality conflicts?

Will we be able to talk to one another, understand our differences, and be tolerant?

What if their way means only one dim light on in the evening or the heat always down to 65 degrees?

Exactly what is important?

Perhaps it is Sunday morning sleep-in time. For many people, this is the only time you feel you can catch up on energy. It might be the only time in the week when you can relax and not feel pressured. Is this wrong?

Many people, including you parents, might say yes. Sunday should be for church. But circumstances, such as working two jobs, may dictate a different way. If your parents might make an issue of this matter, have an agreement about this before you move in together.

Arrange for your parents to go to church. The

church may have a bus pickup. An inquiry might reveal a church member who lives nearby and who is willing to include your parent as an extra passenger. The church may be within walking distance. Walking is the best possible exercise for all ages.

A loving son or daughter will explore every possibility, make arrangements *beforehand,* and occasionally provide the transportation himself or herself. When you do the latter and join your parent at church, you should feel the warmth generated by their appreciation.

Then again, you may be the churchgoer and your father an agnostic curmudgeon. If this is the case, treat him kindly, invite him to go, but do not push your faith. If you display love, concern, and faithfulness, your life may convince him to join you. By our fruits we are known.

You will surprise even yourself if you use well-thought-out, kindly words when discussing controversial situations. Ingrained habits, however, should be considered.

Is your father or mother an early riser? Does he or she like coffee and the news as the day dawns? If this is not your way, buy a small electric percolator, mugs, sugar bowl, and powdered cream, then set up a snack table in your parents' room. Get earphones and ask your parents to use them.

Discuss these things beforehand, too.

Another common question: How will my spouse react to criticism? No matter how careful we are, someone, sometime, will criticize.

When out-of-town guests visit our homes, most of us spruce up the house, caution our children, and cloak ourselves in our best behavior. When the visitors leave, we relax.

If you join forces with parents, will they be like invited guests? Will you feel uneasy as if you are inching through a mine field? Try to act in your usual way, no matter what the consequences.

Perhaps you will need to deal with personal idiosyncrasies. Some of these are common quirks. Every breath of fresh air is a "draft." The fact is, stale air is unhealthy. When you air the house, ask your parents to put on a sweater, sit closer to the heat, find a cozy spot, or withdraw to another room.

Your parent may not drink enough liquids. This causes dehydration and strong-smelling urine. Dr. Moss, in his book, *Caring for the Aged,* suggests drinking two glasses of cranberry juice every day. He says this deodorizes the urine and gets more fluid into the system.

Love will give you insight into many situations. But sometimes love will cause problems.

Some grandparents overindulge their grandchildren. Insist, if necessary, that the older adult understand that you as the parent have the final word. The children should know that you will not tolerate wheedling to get around a decision.

Occasionally these same children, when grown and away from home, may prove a problem. One Christmas Doris' three children as well as the grandchildren descended upon her and her husband. Doris cared for her own bedridden mother and partially blind father. After these children departed, Doris' husband had a heart attack. When things normalized, Doris sat down and wrote a letter. With kindness, she asked her offspring not to come in the future unless she invited them.

In another situation a divorced daughter visited her parents on weekends, dumped her son, then spent all her time telephoning friends and going out with them.

In still another incident, a daughter traveled 500 miles with her children, ostensibly to be there when her mother underwent surgery and to care for her dad. This daughter visited her mother once, cooked nothing for her father, and spent most of the time with a friend. Then the young woman became upset because her father railed at her.

I'm sure it is clear to you that these parents sustained little privacy during these visits and derived little enjoyment from them. Take a tip from this. Be considerate, and when you contemplate living together, think about privacy.

Friends of my parents never thought of joining households when they celebrated their fifty-fifth wedding anniversary. Shortly thereafter both deteriorated physically. Their youngest daughter wanted to keep the families separate but it was to prove impossible.

But neither the parents' house nor the daughter's apartment accommodated the needs of the two families. The daughter's husband and son rose early. They needed a bathroom. The grandparents needed separate bedrooms. But both her apartment and their home had only one bath and two bedrooms. The parents' house, however, had a large attic.

One day the younger couple sat down and presented their suggestions. "What do you think if we leave the downstairs exactly as is for you, and remodel the attic, adding a dormer? A bath can separate the upstairs. Jimmy will move into the smaller area and Bob and I will share the remainder."

"Oh, Denise, how wonderful," her mother said. "Your pa and I worried that we might have to move." The plans provided everyone with a bit of privacy.

Think about specific arrangements you can make for the privacy, safety, and comfort of all generations. One woman placed a television with a remote control in her mother's bedroom. Then she and her husband could entertain, and her mother could watch television or fall asleep whenever she wished. The husband put a second railing on the opposite side of the stairs and a movable barrier at the top. This made climbing the stairs easier and it provided protection against falling down these stairs. He installed safety rails near the toilet and bathtub.

Always consider whatever affords the most privacy. Privacy is important.

Of course, minor and major irritations will arise. When they do, discuss them together and decide to live with them if you cannot remove them.

There is still another potential troublemaker: How do you plan vacations?

Some people take the parents along; some siblings invite the parents; other people hire a "parent-sitter." You might try all three ways at different times. You are not locked in.

Traveling together may disclose facets of your parents that you never knew about or appreciated while growing up. If you leave them at home, they can prove more independent than you expected. In other words, you can solve this dilemma.

There is one decision you must make before you move in together, however, in order to avoid some rocks in life's road. It is the most important decision of all.

Who will be boss?

When you decide this you will also conquer, "Will my parents insist on treating me like their 'little girl' or 'baby boy'?" and "Will they insist we do things their way?" These are some of the questions that make having a boss necessary and require that rules be formulated before the merger.

Outsiders would have said my mother was boss. It wasn't true. She talked everything over with my dad. He usually said, "It's O.K. Do whatever you want." Once in a while, my father disagreed. When this happened, they did it his way.

I was lucky. Mother treated me the same way.

Every household needs a leader. This "boss" should confer with others, respect differing opinions, go along whenever possible; but the final decision should rest squarely on one person's shoulders. The head of your house is the logical maker of the rules.

Be considerate, be kind, show love, and be boss.

You will find that if you ask questions and answer them before consolidating, your lives together should radiate love and your future path be smoother.

You may also discover that nothing you do will ever satisfy your parents. If this should happen, do your best to consider their needs, make your decisions, and then live with them.

6
The Effect on a Marriage

A marriage can split up because of a dependent parent. The anger, like molten lava, may have roiled beneath the surface, but the pressure of an additional dependency may cause the volcano to blow.

Leone considered her ill mother her first priority. She left her husband in a distant state and returned to nurse a mother who died a decade later. The agony of divorce waned as she cared for the house and her parent while her unmarried brother, still living at home, worked and supplied the monetary needs. After the mother's death, when her brother married, Leone was unprepared for other employment. Her age made a job difficult to obtain.

If you face the decision of leaving the security of a marriage to watch over an invalid, consider Leone's predicament.

Besides, in the wedding pledge, didn't you leave mother and father to cleave to your spouse? Your husband or wife is your primary responsibility. And there are solutions to a parent problem that can broaden and deepen the love you share with your spouse. If your mate knows he or she is not usurped by a parent, you inspire cooperation in this spouse.

Cooperation is evident in the second marriage of Nell and Frank. Nell, an only child, knew preparation was important. Before she accepted Frank's proposal, therefore, she explained the possibility of her mother's future need to live with them. Neither Frank nor Nell imagined they would soon be living with two mothers—his as well as hers.

When it became apparent that Frank's sisters

wanted no part of their mother, Nell and Frank took her in. They bought a house with three bedrooms so each mother could have her own room, and they decided never to take sides with either.

Do the mothers get along? Reasonably so. Both complain to their own child, and neither Nell nor Frank agrees with the complainant. Instead, they try to explain the other in-law's behavior.

Does this mean Frank and Nell have no irritations? Of course not. They work each problem out, however, and/or live with it.

Both Nell and Frank plan for times together and alone. In the summer Nell often finds her husband in their travel trailer, reading a book. She lunches with a friend once a week and plays cards regularly with another group. They also bowl or take in a movie. Every Saturday they go to Mass, go out for dinner with friends, and then go to the home of one of their friends.

How do they manage these outings? They employ a "parent-sitter." The mothers protest. But the sitter is there in case of an emergency.

Nell and Frank say, "It's worth every penny we pay the sitters."

Is this paradise? Of course not. After Frank's mother has been in the bathroom, Nell checks and flushes the toilet or turns off the water. She has found it impossible to convince her mother-in-law to do it.

Both admit it resembles living in a nursing home. Her mother is a hypochondriac while his mother is heavy and "throws" herself on the furniture. This keeps Frank busy increasing the supports and fixing broken furniture legs.

Some of these complaints are common in many families. The one mother will not wear a hearing aid. She hears what she wants but rarely responds otherwise. The other mother is legally blind but is able to dress and feed herself. Both are over ninety years old. One mother laughs and jokes; the other does neither. One is generous with her money; the other is frugal.

Nell and Frank insist their mothers pay something. It gives the mothers independence and helps defray the sitter expenses. Nell and Frank also told the mothers they must get along together or they cannot stay.

When the TV selection annoys the mothers, Nell and Frank watch their own choice and let the mothers go to bed or listen with them.

Different problems may come up in the future. I asked Nell, for example, about plans should one or both of the women become bedridden.

"We're not in favor of a nursing home," she said. "We think we'll employ a live-in practical nurse if we face that."

Nell and Frank have also discussed where their parents should be buried since both mothers have plots in distant states. They decided to exchange their own two graves for a four-grave plot.

Nell wonders what will happen to her mother if she herself dies first. She also wonders whether she could cope with Frank's mother if he should die. With the same level-eyed approach she has used to date, however, she says, "There will be a way. I'll cross those bridges when they appear."

This two-mother situation is more common than you think. What will you do if you face it?

You will succeed if you plan ahead, make it understood the parents have to get along, not take sides yourself, and arrange ample time for you and your spouse to do things together or all alone.

You might even say what Nell said to her mother: "You told me what to do for years. Now that you are living in my home, you must follow my requests."

Though parents usually need care after the children are nearing retirement or are retired, it can happen to younger couples who have children at home. When this occurs, how do you keep your parents from reversing your orders and make the money go around?

Once again, set some rules before the generations join and make room for privacy.

If the grandchildren are young when a parent needs a home, explain the situation. Young children understand more than you realize. They can analyze a situation and respond. An eight year old who suffers every time his family moves due to his father's mobility can sympathize with his grandmother who has lost her husband and must change locations. A seven year old can read the mind of the black-coated woman with whom he wishes to share his treasure, a kitten, and say, "The kitten isn't shedding. You won't get hair on your coat."

Your children are just as understanding. They may assess the situation whether or not you explain. Clue them in, however, then trust them to understand. You may find their opinion is your salvation.

My mother told me she would never have weathered the Great Depression if it had not been for my childish faith. "God will take care of us," I would tell her. And He did. A little child may lead you to serenity through his or her perception.

Tell your children before the generations join and ask for cooperation. You may need to remind them from time to time, but they can prove to be your biggest helpers. Children usually like grandparents.

Explain to your parents. Make them understand that when you punish or encourage your children, they are not to disapprove in front of the children. Your parents may discuss their differences with you, but they should do that in private; and advise them that you may not agree. (Should you see the wisdom of their private advice, however, do not be too proud to acknowledge it or to do differently.)

The husband's parents living with you can be a trial to a wife, especially if this wife must care for young children. When this is the situation, use some of Nell and Frank's ideas.

The wife's parents may prove a financial drain on the husband. He may resent this while trying to raise a family. In situations like this, can the wife take a part-time job? Can some kind of work be carried on at home? Perhaps the dependent mother has a talent. Can she help out by performing tasks like shortening hems? Many small dress shops welcome an expert at this sort of thing and will deliver and pick up the garments.

A handiwork expert might direct that ability to making paraments for the altars of churches or special stoles for ministers. One day I commented on the unusual stole a pastor wore. He told me how it, and others, were specially designed for him by a talented older woman. Perhaps your mother or mother-in-law can make some extra money by using her skills.

Maybe you or the parent can be a member of an arts and crafts store or novelty shop and sell handmade articles on consignment.

Men sometimes build bird feeders or suet holders and create woodcarvings, shelves, and magazine racks. Can your male parent find a market for some of his work?

A senior co-op store in Santa Cruz, California, charges a dollar per year for dues and takes a percentage of the price received on items sold. The co-op also requires a specific number of hours of work. One man is so adept at making toys, building blocks, and cut-out numbers that during one November alone, he cleared $1,200. This co-op also has an annex for antiques. Many people dispose of treasures through this section.

A financial problem will not be as great if your parent has a money-making interest he or she is willing to pursue. Discuss this before the merger.

Once again, do think about vacations. My friend's family always camped out. When my friend was eleven, her grandmother came to live with them. The grandmother was adamant about their taking her on their vacations. Yet the grandmother could not breathe well in higher elevations. Nor could she rest in a sleeping bag, hike on trails, or leave the comforts of an inside bathroom. My friend remembers how upset she became when their camping trips ceased. She resented her grandmother.

Don't take the same kind of vacation year after year. Nell and Frank use the parent-sitter for weekends when they shop or go to the theater in a nearby city. Your family must have some time away from the older generation, if at all possible. And your parents in turn need time away from you and yours.

Sometimes this is not feasible. Suppose the older person is seriously ill, or you have had an unexpected expense. Explain the reasons to your children. Try to arrange something as an acceptable substitute. They may be upset at the moment, but explanations can avoid a buildup of frustration or hatred.

Make allowances so you and your spouse can enjoy a private vacation. You may return with renewed love for your spouse.

Just as you need vacations apart, you should continue to entertain in your home. Privacy arrangements for each member of the family will help you in this.

It is not advantageous to include all occupants of your home in every entertainment plan. Suppose your children want some kind of party. If you think the noise will annoy your parents, make plans for them to spend the night at the home of one of their other children or relative or close friend. Your parents need outside activities, too.

Arrange for special nights when your parents

invite friends. You can help them prepare, or you can get out of the house—whatever your parents want. Let your children know it is gramps' or grandma's night.

In November 1978, *Good Housekeeping* magazine printed an article called, "My Husband and I Could Never Be Alone." The author and her husband looked forward to exciting times after their children married and left home. The author's father died, however, and they took in her desolate mother. Shortly thereafter, when their daughter's marriage broke up, the daughter also moved in with them, got a job, and expected her mother to baby-sit. This ended any aloneness for the couple.

Then on their wedding anniversary, Hal announced he had arranged a three-week vacation. "It's impossible," his wife said. "Mother would be helpless. Who would take care of our grandchild?"

"Well, if you can't, I can. . . . I'm going. I can learn to manage without you. The things is . . . I don't want to. Will you go?"

"Yes," his wife replied.

When they returned, they discovered the mother had made her own social plans and their daughter had found a teenaged girl to baby-sit.

You can break ties, too. The Bible tells us to bear one another's burdens, but it also says everyone should carry his or her own burden. The secret is to know when to do which.

Another form of cooperation is the grandparent/grandchild relationship. Most children want a grandparent. They love and trust these older people.

In May 1981, *Newsweek* wrote about a new book, *Grandparents/Grandchildren, The Vital Connection.* This book argues that today's grandchildren are big losers because TV, day-care centers, and paperback books are taking over for grandparents. The authors of this book, Arthur Kornhaber and Kenneth L. Woodward, say,

"Grandparents and grandchildren do not have to do anything to make each other happy. . . . Happiness comes from being together."

Grandparents can smooth out tense situations in which you are caught in the middle. Their presence in your home can mean a happier marriage for you and a positive influence on your children, if you will allow it to happen.

Sometimes marriage problems arise because of money. One couple insisted the wife's mother divide her assets when she moved in with them. She did. The daughter and husband enlarged their home with their half of the assets. This mother is now in her nineties; she is able to get around and is mentally alert. The daughter never expected her mother would live so long and screams that someday she will sell the house and toss her mother out on the street. Yet when the son, whose home is very small, suggests a nursing home, the daughter refuses to consider it.

Does your mother have peace of mind if she lives with one of your sisters or brothers? Do you? What can you do if you feel a parent is being abused?

Most states have a Department of Human Services, and included in this department is an Office of the Aging. Employees in this office can advise sons and daughters of the rights available when parent abuse is discovered. If you call 1-800-555-1212, you will get the free telephone number for this service in the state in which your parent resides.

For many reasons, a son or daughter is wise in not touching the parents' money. Some parents who distribute their assets become suspicious of what has happened to it. Sometimes they demand a return. Sometimes it is important to obtain power of attorney so you can use this money for the aid of your parents.

If you ever feel your parent is being abused, you have recourse. In Arkansas, and in other states, the

Protective Services Unit is responsible for the implementation of Act 166 (Ark. Stat. Ann. 59-1301). (See appendix for what this includes.)

In Arkansas the Office on Aging has a Protective Services Unit consisting of four Protective Services Consultants and one Secretary under the supervision of the Legal Services Development Specialist.

Reports of suspected adult abuse are referred to the Central Registry via a WATS line or a toll-free line. If any legal action is warranted, the Protective Services Consultant, in conjunction with the Office on Aging Legal Services Development Specialist, will prepare and present the case. This, of course, is after an investigation has been made. The act covers all adults.

Did you know that abuse of an adult can be considered a Class D felony and punished by law? A person is guilty who willfully or by culpable negligence deprives an adult of necessary food, clothing, shelter, or medical treatment; or who allows an adult to be so deprived; or who is knowingly guilty of negligence that permits the physical or mental health of the adult to be materially endangered.

The main purpose of the law is to protect adults unable to protect themselves. Anyone with reasonable cause to suspect that an adult is being abused may report this (see appendix for instructions).

The Arkansas law, and maybe the one in your state, has not been advertised. Those who know of it learned by word of mouth. It was first enacted by the Arkansas State Legislature in 1977.

When the law was first enacted, the state personnel expected to handle about 300 cases per year with only five percent of these being substantiated. In the first five months of operation, approximately 320 cases were opened, and nearly twenty percent were verified.

If you suspect abuse, report it for investigation. It is more prevalent than you realize.

Counsel with your brothers and sisters early on if you feel you are becoming frustrated and may endanger your marriage and your parent. There is a way out.

Another factor that can produce strain on your marriage is the physical illness of one or both of your parents. If your parent lives with you, you may be shocked some morning. The person standing in the doorway may look like a stranger. One side of the mouth may droop; one hand may dangle; one foot may be turned in a peculiar fashion; eyes may try to tell you what the voice no longer can.

This possibility is why, several years before my mother-in-law's stroke, we had added the dormer and bath to our upstairs—in case she needed to live with us.

Dr. Moss, in his *Caring for the Aged,* suggests putting stroke victims where they can continue to watch life around them. This provides mental stimulus. He also advises against institutionalization.

Today there are home health care agencies to help you. Just yesterday I sat in a volunteer session of our hospice organization and heard men planning to visit the homes of several stroke victims to rig up a "contraption" that would provide therapy for them.

Look around your home. Is there some change you can make that will be useful to you now and yet prove to be a cozy spot for a dependent parent, ill or not?

There is help available for you so you can care for a physically ill parent in your home, if you so desire.

Discuss this with your spouse. We are told that communication is one of the keys to a happy marriage. It is even more important when that marriage might be threatened by the needs of aging parents.

Keep the lines of communication open. Be optimistic. And use your pipeline to God. He can help you solve all your problems. Doesn't His Word say, "Cast your cares on the Lord and he will sustain you" (Psalm 55:22)?

7
Is a Care Facility Necessary?

Old age can be a sorry time. The Preacher in Ecclesiastes tells us our hands and legs will tremble, we will be bowed down, our eyes will see less, our ears will hear less, we will stop chewing for lack of teeth, and we will awaken at early morning to the voice of a bird.

How will you feel when you see the powers of your parents fading? How will you feel if you must entrust them to the care of others?

It is often true that as people age, two systems— the physical and the mental—may deteriorate in varying degrees. When mental or physical capabilities wane, your choices may be limited.

Should you continue to try to care for your parents at home (theirs or yours) or should you place them in a nursing home? Your heart says keep them. What does your head say?

Again, there are questions to answer.

A. How do you decide when a care facility is necessary?
B. What are the advantages of a care facility?
C. How do you choose a facility?
D. How is your parent protected?
E. What can you do if you become concerned about the facility after it is chosen?
F. How do you gain your parent's cooperation?
Let's look at each of these questions in turn.

A. How do you decide when a care facility is necessary?

Dr. Linden, whom I quoted earlier, says three occasions make a care facility necessary.

1. When physical illness needs attention.

2. When your parents cannot care for themselves.

3. When instruments, treatments, and programs of care that a private home does not have are needed.

Dr. Linden says, "A child's love . . . no matter how great . . . does not take the place of good medical care."

Some consolation for you as you answer this question is contained in an issue of "Your Retirement Advisor," a four-page pamphlet prepared for various companies to mail to their retired employees. It stated that only five percent of older people require nursing home care. Does this surprise you? It did me.

But think about this possibility. Be truthful with yourself and your parent. One wise question to ask is: If the parent remains with me, can I cope?

Florence relied on her retired husband to "sit" with her mother. One morning the husband was rushed to the hospital. He died that week.

Later, when Florence's mother entered a hospital for tests, the doctor advised moving her to a nursing facility. "It will be easier for her to adjust," he said, "and if I move her now, you needn't worry about a waiting list."

The daughter paced the floor. If she entered her mother, would she be doing it for her mother's sake or for her own?

Physical disability often takes a specific kind of nursing, but how can you tell if a person is emotionally disturbed and in need of institutional care? You can be suspicious if several things become noticeable.

Does your parent suddenly disown a child for no logical reason? Has your parent come to believe that normal activity is not worth the effort?

Some aging adults act like children, believe they are persecuted, or become hypochondriacs. This does not mean they are mentally disturbed.

Be kind as you watch your parents. Do not believe

that every deviation from what you consider normal is a bad sign.

Perhaps your parents have decided they are old enough to stop putting up a front. Maybe they have determined to do only those things they really *want* to do.

If you believe in God, pray about your doubts before acting. If your parent is deeply depressed or mentally unstable, however, insist on an appointment with a physician. If at all possible, go with your parent. Talk to the doctor. Ask questions.

Medication may cause slurring of speech, hallucinations, and mental unrest. It happened to Justice Rehnquist. The doctor may be able to prescribe a medicine that will produce no side effects for your parent. Find out if the medication is at fault or if your parent is deteriorating.

Perhaps the medication is being taken at an improper time. When is the right time? If your parent has a favorite food, this could cause a wrong interaction.

Sometimes the reactions of your own children may alert you to the failing of your parent.

As one grandmother slipped both physically and mentally, she would unbutton her dress while her grandson's friends lounged nearby. She was not aware of the visitors or the hour.

Though this grandmother had two daughters, Greta, the mother of the sons, kept her more than six months each year. One day Greta answered the phone and heard: "I can't keep mother any longer." The sister calling had previously refused to consider institutional care.

Greta hated to refuse. Her husband explained it was disturbing the life of their children and becoming too big a burden for Greta.

"Let's pray about it," said Greta.

They drove to the nursing home where they often volunteered their services, but the administrator said, "I'm sorry. We have no beds. I'll have to put her on a list."

The day the sister was to arrive at Greta's house with their mother, the nursing home administrator called Greta and said, "If you can bring your mother today, we can take her." Greta says that never in her life has she felt more certain something was right. Nor can she remember ever receiving a quicker answer to prayer.

Did you know that God's eyes run to and fro throughout the whole earth to show Himself strong in our behalf? (2 Chronicles 16:9). He answers. Sometimes He uses split-second timing!

B. What are the advantages of a care facility?

They can be many: regular hours, a balanced diet, medical help available at all times, the assurance that medications are taken as prescribed, and rehabilitation therapy, if needed.

But there are also needs of the heart. These should be supplied by the parent's relatives.

Sometimes the parent may keep asking to go home. In one instance, the daughter brought her mother to her house for the afternoon. Soon this mother said, "They'll miss me at dinner. I'd better go back."

Your mother or father may react the same way. There is fellowship around a dining room table and plenty of activities for residents. Many church groups worship with nursing home residents. Soloists (like me) give mini-concerts. Youth choirs, bell-ringers, and vocal ensembles bring special music. Community players perform or give bingo parties with a banana as a prize.

In a nursing facility your parent can attend interesting events that would otherwise be impossible to attend. Sometimes he or she may even renew old acquaintances. My mother's cousin found another cousin in the home she entered.

Check the roster. See if a friend of your parent lives there. Having a friend who has chosen to enter a certain care facility may convince your parent that it is O.K. for him or her too.

Once you decide your parent needs institutional care, you may wonder how you find a good home.

C. How do you choose a facility?

According to the Citizens for Better Nursing Home Care, Inc., located in Santa Cruz, California, it will be to your advantage to get adequate information about care facilities even before it is needed. But circumstances may not enable you to do so.

The Mid-Coast Comprehensive Health Planning Association researched and wrote a guide entitled, *Nursing Home and Alternative Care.* This guide answers questions about the available services. Your ombudsman/advocate can give you current information on local long-term care facilities.

Some places are better than others, and different ones have special strengths. Investigate each facility.

My husband and I did this when his mother was hospitalized with her second stroke. My mother-in-law was not in a position to choose, but if your parent can, involve him or her in the choice.

Read the contract carefully. Ask questions.

The daily rate charged by the nursing home does not always cover all costs. Be aware of extra charges. Keep a copy of the contract for the home you feel is best. The way to find this home is to research the area by obtaining the names of as many nursing homes as possible. To compile this list, contact your local health department, medical society, hospital or nursing association, senior citizens' or social work groups, and the social security district office in your community. Physicians, clergy, relatives, and friends will pass on advice.

Before making your choice, be sure to discuss your parents' future with their personal physician. The doctor can advise what kind of home is best since there are differences.

Then use the telephone. Call each place. Rules differ. The information you gain will help you eliminate homes from your list.

After you discover which ones offer the services your parent requires, inspect them and speak with the administrators. First visit the ones most convenient for family visits and closest to a hospital.

The Illinois Council for Long-Term Care has compiled a list that will help you choose wisely (see the appendix). When you have answered the questions on this list, you will know which facility will be best. But before your decision is final, ask one more question.

D. How is your parent protected?

You will want to know this because after your parent is admitted, you may receive a call from one of the personnel saying, "Your parent is missing."

In a two-year period in Chicago, 1,618 men and 802 women over age sixty-five disappeared from various kinds of homes. What does the institution where you propose to take your parent do to prevent this?

Some administrators give the front door guards pictures of the potential runaways. These guards try to persuade the people to remain inside. In a good home, personnel are aware of potential trouble.

Most people who stroll from the grounds are found within twenty-four hours. But others believe $300 a month is better than $25 or $30 and successfully seek another address. Social Security officials under the Federal Privacy Act are not permitted to reveal this address. But if your parent is smart enough to leave the home, discover a new place and arrange for receiving a social security check, he or she probably does not belong in such a facility. You may have to rethink what is best for your parent.

For the parents who just wander but become repeaters, try to find out why. Is it inactivity? People who have led a busy life rebel at sitting around useless. Does it appear to be a legitimate complaint against the care, food, or administration of the facility?

If the reasons involve the management, try to work this out with the administrator. If you are not successful, contact your ombudsman program. The Comprehensive Older Americans Act Amendments of 1978 require every state to have such a program.

What is an ombudsman program? The program provides objective, unbiased, reconciliatory mediators whose goals are to improve and maintain the quality of life for nursing home patients. They have established ways to receive and resolve complaints. They document significant problems of long-term care. They inform the public of the realities of nursing homes and promote increased understanding and awareness of these problems.

If your parent is upset by some situation and the ombudsman representative is informed, the authenticity of the complaint will be checked. The complainant always receives a report of the results of the evaluation.

Remember that this is an objective, unbiased group. If the home is at fault, the group will tell you and advise you of the steps that will be taken to correct the situation. If your parent is being unjust, you will also learn this.

In Santa Cruz, California, they established a volunteer in each facility. These volunteers receive ombudsman training.

When a complaint is received by telephone, mail, or as a result of the direct outreach of the ombudsman, action is initiated immediately. This service is free and offers strict confidentiality.

Many problems are solved quickly. If necessary, however, the problem may be referred to State Licensing or to the state ombudsman for final settlement. When a situation is solved satisfactorily, the local ombudsmen make follow-up visits to be sure it does not recur.

This knowledge should set your mind at ease about your parent's residency in these homes.

The Comprehensive Older Americans Act Amendments of 1978 strengthened the ombudsman program considerably, giving the program explicit statutory authority. Ombudsman functions and responsibilities are defined, and the program's concern has been broadened to *all* long-term care facilities.

Do not hesitate to contact your ombudsman representative, and be aware of the kinds of homes available. You may wish to move your parents. Change is possible no matter what kind of home was chosen originally.

Some churches administer retirement homes, such as Pilgrim Haven in Los Altos, California, and Bethany Home and Hospital in Chicago. Many of these have rooms and apartments, communal dining rooms, and medical and nursing care. Board-and-care homes and residential care homes are available. In these the residents have rooms and are given meals. Fraternal organizations usually have facilities for the aged. All these are in addition to regular nursing homes and convalescent hospitals.

Some states have a new development that allows the elderly to live together in private residences. Massachusetts has foster care for the elderly.

The Superintendent of Documents, U.S. Government Printing Office, Washington, D.C. 20402, can supply you with many helpful booklets. Some are free. Mail order is not the only way to get these. Sixteen states, plus the District of Columbia, have bookstores in which you can browse through the shelves for what you want. With all these possibilities, you should find information to help you pick the proper facility, if your parent needs it.

Once your parent is a resident of a home, there is another question to ask.

E. What can you do personally if you are concerned about your parent's treatment?

This question excludes the ombudsman program and involves projects you can spark to help in the treatment given.

In one community, relatives and friends discovered that the nursing home cooks were unable to prepare nutritious meals. A group of these concerned people approached the local school and asked if a special course could be provided for the cooks. A nutritionist agreed to teach such a course. Now the confined parents are fed adequately. Perhaps you, too, can spearhead a drive to get a nutrition course set up for your parents' chefs, if it is necessary.

You might encourage good care by giving an Aide of the Year Award. This would recognize those who provide exceptional care and show concern for the comfort and dignity of the patients.

You might also determine whether your state has a Patients' Rights List. If not, write for a summary of S.N.F.R. Section 72523 of the California Health and Safety Code. Work through your ombudsman so your parent and others will be aware of their personal rights.

Sometimes you would like a change in your parent's attitude regarding entering a home.

F. How do you gain your parent's cooperation?

Many of us do not want to see our parents among such a group. We struggle with mixed emotions before we accept it.

Most people resist going. Somehow, for nearly all of us, there is a stigma attached to what some people call "an old people's home."

If the reason your parent enters a nursing home is that instruments, treatments, and programs of care are needed, you should find this the easiest to explain. Be sure your parents know you are not putting them into a nursing home to get rid of them. If there is a possibility they will improve enough to return to their previous location, tell them so. It may encourage them to make progress.

If you have discovered that one of your parent's friends lives in the home, say so. It may be the key to unlocking the door of your parent's resistance.

If your parent likes parties, emphasize the activities and birthday parties that are held regularly. Your parent might decide attending would prove better than sitting alone.

There is also the old adage I remember from my childhood: "Prayer changes things." It does, you know. In fact, it should be the first, not the last, thing you try when attempting to change the mind of a resistant parent.

Above all, be sincere, show your love, convince your parent you are doing this for his or her good. These feelings can be read in your expression, your tone of voice, and the words you choose. Your parent will sense your attitude and be more willing to consider a nursing home as an option.

8
An Hour or a Day?

How much time do you *owe* your parent or parents? What portion of your life do you *wish* to share?

Loving children want to help a parent. We need not feel guilty, however, if we do not do everything demanded of us.

Gwen had married recently. Her father died shortly after the wedding. Every morning her mother appeared at her new home, and every evening the mother expected Gwen to walk home with her and spend the night. Naturally, it began to affect the new marriage.

If your mother drops in often and demands too much of your time, there are some things you can try. They may or may not work.

First, discuss the problem openly and truthfully. Ask your parent for ideas, too. Do you have a special time to vacuum, dust, and straighten the house? Do you plan free time for a luncheon date, a church gathering, neighborhood coffee? If so, tell your parent. Ask for cooperation.

Second, just as you save time for your other outings, set aside time for your parent. Give your loved one your complete attention during that period.

Have you ever thought that they may be grabbing any time they can because you don't really listen to them? You may be so involved in things you believe *must* be done that you think you cannot spare a second. Take time. Remember, people are more important than things. You will be better for the relaxing break, and you will discover your relations with these loved ones will improve.

Third, plan a surprise or buy some handwork you can do together. My cousin has become an excellent needle-pointer because he was forced to curtail more active pursuits. I proudly show the pillow he made for me. Your parent, like him, may even go on to designing original patterns on graph paper and working them out.

Learn a new game, preferably one your parents can play alone or with just one other partner. Suggest and hand them a book you have read and enjoyed.

If a meeting you attend regularly is open for all ages, invite your mother. If your children are performing or playing an athletic game, take your parents. You may get a surprise. Grandchildren love to have grandparents watch them.

My youngest grandson is not athletic but he was on a Peewee League team. One day my strikeout leader hit a triple. Afterward, munching on the hot dog his manager bought him, he confessed he didn't know how he did it. "I was as surprised as anybody, grandma," he said. But both of us knew he was glad I had been there to see it.

If you work outside the home, save an evening for your parents and call in-between times. There are considerate ways to terminate a telephone conversation if it threatens to become lengthy. Perhaps the oven bell rings, you have to put up the hem on a daughter's dress so she can wear it that night, or you may have promised a neighbor you would run some errand. You may even have to go to the bathroom. If you wish, tell your parent you will call back later. When you tell a parent this, however, keep your promise.

Be kind and calm. Encourage your parents to find hobbies, friends, activities, and outings that relieve you while enhancing their enjoyment of life.

Constantly chauffeuring and running errands can eat into your time. It can hinder your husband—be he son or son-in-law—from fixing the leaking faucet in your own house. If parents make demands on his time, suggest he allocate a certain evening, or day, to caring for their problems. This arrangement can protect marital harmony because no spouse wishes to slip into second place, and no wife enjoys the procrastination of a husband. In most instances, cooperation can be obtained if parents know there will always be time for them.

One daughter in our town, a widow herself, designates a specific day when she takes her mother and mother-in-law shopping. They return books to the library, look for a new comforter or sweater, or replenish their larders. She is on call if a medical emergency arises, of course, but for a physical checkup or something not requiring haste, she asks them to schedule it on the day she receives her allergy shot.

Does she neglect these widows at other times? Not at all. They often share meals, attend some special program, or talk on the telephone.

Help your parent willingly, but do not allow this parent to impose upon you unjustly, even if he or she is sometimes lonesome.

When I was a young service representative for the telephone company, I discovered that some elderly people called the business office because they wanted to talk to someone—anyone. This may be true of your parents. What can you do about it?

Perhaps you can arrange for a friend to call. If your mother or father does not attend your church, see if the one they go to has any activity made accessible for older people by bus service. Some churches provide a ride for those interested in attending special events. Encourage your parents to join in. Check on the services for the aging in your county and see if any arrange some activity in which your parents would find new friends and dispel some of their loneliness.

Do your parents expect to be invited to every

party you give? If they are not included, are they offended? Ask them on certain occasions. When you do not wish them to join you, give them a detailed rundown of what happened and any other tidbits of interest. Make them feel as if they were present. This should not only assuage any hurt feelings but also give them fuel for conversations with friends. Nearly all parents like to talk about their children.

If your parents live far from you, call or write to keep them aware of the happenings in the life of your family. Dear Abby included in her column a letter from a woman who visits her "sometimes senile" mother at the convalescent home every day but whose sisters and brothers cannot stand the smell or become too depressed. Dear Abby has also printed letters from normal mothers whose sons live next door or ten minutes away yet visit only once a month for five minutes and never cut the grass, paint, or even talk. Don't be like either of these types.

One daughter visited her institutionalized mother every day for ten years. Think of it. She and her husband never took a vacation and never went out of town.

You may be different. You may dread visiting your parent and, as a result, seldom do so. You may also wonder, *What can we talk about?*

One younger woman did an excellent job with a mother who seemed to be totally oblivious to all the world about her. This young woman sat by her mother's bedside, held her hand (touching is important), and told her about the weather, the cardinals raising a family in the arborvitae in front of her window, her pratfall on slippery mud, and little items about her family and friends. One day many months after the daughter began these unanswered conversations, her mother struggled to say something. Out of a strained throat, in a raspy, quivery voice, came the words "I love you."

What a reward!

So talk. Talk about anything that interests you—the old days, memories, or today.

Bring presents. You may discover that theft is often prevalent in nursing homes. Marked gowns, socks, and robes are lost in the laundry. Replenish these with little surprise packages. A parent may delight, like a child, in opening a gift. Once in a while bring a single rose or a small bottle of cologne. An ice cream cone, a sundae, or a Hershey bar may also bring a smile.

An elderly friend, a second mother to me, lives far away. The other night I called her. As we talked, she mentioned one of my best friends who had been in Chicago and had phoned her. When we ended our call, she said, "I always thank God for you and Cindy [the girl who called] and Ilsa. You girls call me and write to me much more than my own grandchildren."

The length of time we spend with our parents is not necessarily as important as the frequency of our contact. Though organizations like the Telephone Pioneers of America thoughtfully visit more than some sons and daughters, it is not the same.

"Friendship is crucial for life," said Dr. James F. Drane in a column in the *Arkansas Gazette.* Yes, adults need friends, but they also need family.

It is true that institutionalized people are not always easy to visit. In fact, some may never have anyone call because of the fuss they make. We children, in turn, get caught up in activities. Then suddenly we realize we have neglected our parents. No matter what distance you live from your parents, no matter whether they reside with a relative, by themselves, or in a home, try to contact them at least once a week.

When you visit hospitalized parents, don't worry whether they are aware of you or of any gift you may take. Don't be upset if they forget. You will know you cared.

If possible, take your parent out for a ride or for a shopping jaunt, or wheel or walk them around the grounds of the home. One grandson visited his institutionalized grandmother faithfully. As he pushed her wheelchair to a ramp and gave it a gentle shove, the grandmother giggled with glee. When he retrieved her, she had a lively twinkle in her eye.

"Most older people do . . . well, if somebody talks to them," says Dr. Linden. "If you talk to them they begin to sparkle. . . . Touching is important. . . . Touching conveys . . . feeling."

Berit Scott, writing in *Ladies' Home Journal,* said her invalid mother surprised her on one visit by leaning her head in Berit's direction and closing her eyes instead of staring wide-eyed and unseeing. Berit patted her mother's shoulder awkwardly, kissed her forehead and said, "I'll be back soon. . . . I love you, Mother."

Medical personnel encourage us to speak to people in a coma. Whisper words of love. Give a touch of endearment. These may ease the spirit of an unseeing, uncommunicative parent.

It is important to keep in touch with your parents, no matter how unnoticing they may be and no matter where they live.

Also, keep your promises. A lovely elderly woman remembered that one of her daughters promised to come 200 miles and get her on Christmas Day. Early that morning she let her other daughter help her pack her bags. The mother waited and waited. After 10:00 P.M. she finally gave in and went to bed. Keep your promises. If you live at a distance, even a card with a few words like "Luv ya" is welcome.

One woman found letters a partial solution when visits to her hospitalized, belligerent mother became a draining experience. Each day this woman mails her mother a "bulletin." She types six different bulletins at a time and includes news of the family, comments on life, and omits any bad news. She uses uppercase letters and double spacing. It takes about an hour a week, she says. This is a small price to pay to show love. She continues to visit occasionally and finds the visits are now more pleasant.

Even if you live close to your parents, you can surprise them with mail. My mother and I lived together, but this never stopped me from sending her a card I saw as I searched for ones for my friends.

After my mother's death, I found one of these cards in her Bible. It was dog-eared and tear-splotched but treasured. I had paid 35¢ or 50¢ for it when most cards were a dime. The verse started out:

This morning when I wakened
And saw the sun above,
I softly said, "Good Morning, Lord
—Bless everyone I love!"
Right away I thought of you. . . .

Plan some surprises for your loved ones. It's worth it.

Telephone calls are more personal than cards or letters. If you don't feel like writing, call. "It's the next best thing to being there," the Bell System told us.

Suggest exchanging tapes. Your parents can hear your voice and can share so much. They may not tell you how painful it is to write with their arthritic fingers. They may not realize dimming eyesight is the reason scribbling a letter is not as much fun as it used to be. A tape may be the answer.

Even if you follow none of the above ideas, please remember your parents on Mother's Day, Father's Day, their birthdays, Valentine's Day, Easter, and Christmas. You can be sure most of them will show your lovely card or gift to everyone and brag about how wonderful you are.

If you send or take gifts on these days, and I hope

you will, be selective. A magazine subscription may be well received. Many magazines are now published in large print. When you get Publisher's Clearing House sweepstakes letters, don't throw them away. See what bargains they are offering. They also straighten out any problems and handle changes of address.

Some parents traveled when they were able. A picturesque travel magazine or one of the regional publications like *Arizona Highways* or *Vermont Life* could put wings on their rocking chairs and stir their memories.

You can bring or send fruit. Be sure your parent can eat it, however. This past Christmas a friend had to send home with her son all the fruit she received. She can no longer digest it.

Sweet-smelling lotions or bath oils can be good gifts. Special soaps for men are now available. I would suggest you first try out the item you propose to give since some might prove too slippery.

Have you thought about giving your father a tray with legs? It can be used either for eating in bed or as a holder for books, games, writing equipment, or whatever. You might give him a remote-control station-changer for the TV set. A new record or tape can provide hours of entertainment. Have you seen the Swiss Army knives? Their versatility is unique. Many even include an ivory toothpick.

Gifts are great, but your presence is even more welcome.

The following is an extreme example, but I had a friend who after her marriage drove a twenty-mile round trip each day to help her mother keep up the big house the mother refused to sell. Ultimately, the children convinced their mother to sell the house, but my friend continued to check her daily.

While my husband's mother worked, she lived about sixty-five miles from us. We called her often and invited her to visit whenever she had weekends off. When she relinquished her job but remained independent, she moved fifteen miles nearer to us. We continued inviting her and also arranged to drive out immediately after church at least one Sunday a month. We took her to dinner, then returned to her place for a cozy visit.

Only you can decide how much time to share with your parent. Most parents are long-suffering; they love you and are proud of you. They are satisfied with very little return on the investment they made in your upbringing. Why not emulate God? He gives full measure, pressed down, and running over.

Through our visits we will know our parents better. We will be aware of their interests and their needs. We can take them to a play, concert, or special eating place for a birthday instead of giving them another slip or tie to add to the twenty-five they now own but never wear.

One Christmas Day mother and I did not exchange gifts. She had been in the hospital for six weeks and had returned home the week before the holiday to continue recuperating. That morning, after I changed her bed and bathed her, she looked up at me and said, "Maxine, you're so good to me. Someday I'll make it up to you."

The tears are even now in my eyes as I remember my reply on that day before she died. I said, "Mother, you don't owe me anything. You paid in advance for all this tender loving care."

Isn't that true?

Our parents don't owe us. We owe them—for many things, tangible and intangible, like shelter and food, convictions and character.

We can return a little interest on their investment if we lay aside a little of our time for them.

9
Overcoming Hazards

We provide nourishment of the soul by our consideration of our parents, but physical independence is equally important.

Some parents adamantly refuse to see a doctor. "I'm all right," my father always said. But he wasn't. Only after he was brought home from work, never to return, did he agree to see a doctor. Because I was not even eighteen years old myself, I never thought of the necessity for regular checkups, either.

But you must. Arrange for your parents to have checkups with doctors, dentists, and ophthalmologists.

Today, doctors say that a yearly physical examination is not essential for everyone. If your physician agrees, encourage only the occasional checkup. If possible, go with your parents. Though they may not admit it, they may feel more secure and comfortable if you come along. If you accompany them, you may learn helpful information for the future.

This may be the proper time to advise the doctor of the erratic driving habits of your parents. Do they ignore stoplights and speed limits? Do they drive so slowly they are a menace?

Many states require regular testing after age seventy-two. Some, like Arkansas, have no eye examination. If you feel your parents are endangering themselves and others, take them to the ophthalmologist or the family practitioner. An examination may confirm your suspicions. Then exert loving pressure on your parents.

The child of an elderly man I know arranged for other couples to pick up her parents when going to the same meetings. One day she discovered her father's driving license was close to expiration. She took him for the test. He did not pass. If you know driving is a problem, step in.

Uncle Walt, in the comic strip Gasoline Alley, passed his test and then forgot where he left the car! The test itself is not necessarily the only criterion for qualified driving.

Another issue you may want to talk about with the doctor is your parents' eating habits. If their eating habits are bad, alert the doctor. His word may impress your parents more than yours.

When the doctor prescribes medication, ask him to suggest ways to assure these drugs are taken properly. Perhaps counting them out in the morning and placing them in a specific place will provide the solution. Researchers at the Harvard Medical School and the Massachusetts Institute of Technology have designed an electronic pill vial cap. It can be preset to sound a signal and flash a light when a dose is due. The Med-Tymer, as it is called, resets itself every time the cap is removed and shows if the battery is still strong. It can be set to issue this alarm only during waking hours. If these procedures are made habits, over- or under-medication can be avoided.

One blind woman is still sharp enough to take her pills on time. She distinguishes one pill from another by asking the druggist to put the pills in different kinds of bottles that she places in a particular order.

If your parents wear glasses, instruct them to put these on before reaching for their drugs. This should ensure their taking the right medicine with the proper frequency.

When you visit your parents, look for hazards in their home.

Bathrooms are dangerous places. See that hand-rails are installed. My eighty-year-old neighbor plans to get rid of the metal hold-onto that clamps over the side of the tub. She has discovered a permanent rail is better.

Remove the shining smoothness from the bottom of the bathtub by attaching decals or providing a mat. Show your parents how to step onto every part of that mat before lowering themselves into the water. If they do this, the suction holds better.

Can a shower stall be provided? This is safer than a tub. Or purchase one of the flexible-tubed, hand-held shower heads. With this a person can stand, wet the body, soap all over, and then rinse. Most faucets adapt to this attachment.

Is there a portable electric heater in the bathroom? If so, remove it. Portable heaters can prove to be hazardous. A wet towel or facecloth can be dropped on it. Retrieving these might result in an electric shock. A person could trip, fall on a portable heater, and be burned. A robe or nightgown could ignite if it is too close to a hot heater. Instead, make other arrangements for warmth. You could, for instance, rewire the room to include one or two warming bulbs in the ceiling.

Arrange for permanently lit nightlights in the bathroom and hall. Put a similar fixture in the bedroom or suggest a flashlight on the night table. Some flashlights are small yet easy for even an arthritic hand to grip.

Should your physically fit mother or father wish to wash the walls or paint, fine. But please don't let him or her tackle the ceilings. Employ a professional or donate your own services.

When you visit your parent, look at the furniture and appliances. Bulbs in floor lamps, table lamps, and lower hanging fixtures are changed more easily than those in the ceiling.

Most of us drag over a chair when the bulb in a high fixture must be replaced. We don't bother to get a stepstool. We gamble that we will not fall and break a bone. Try to eliminate this hazard.

Be sure there are no trailing cords. Buy some clips, anchor the cords to the walls, or wind them on a safety shortener.

Place light switches at the top and bottom of stairways. If a hall is more than several feet, have a switch at both ends.

Just as it may be necessary for an electrician to install replacement outlets or switches, so it may be necessary to replace worn out appliances. When a new refrigerator is necessary, look at ones with the freezer on the bottom. No one gets into or cleans the freezer as often as the refrigerator part. When the freezer is on the bottom, refrigerated items in the back or on the bottom shelf are easier to reach. This kind is also more economical than the side-by-side kind.

The proper stove can eliminate dangers, too. There are models that have upper ovens with doors opening upward and over. This helps eliminate bending against a hot door or burning an elbow. Some stoves include an oven burner coil that is removable for easy cleaning.

Try to provide low-level storage space and up-and-down shelves in one end of the closet rather than in overhead ones.

Please remove scatter rugs. Older people often shuffle and fail to pick up their feet. It is easier to stumble if scatter rugs are used.

Discourage your parent from waxing floors. If your mother likes a high gloss, ask her to install one of the no-wax vinyls, or treat her and have it laid yourself.

If your parent likes to wear bedroom slippers, dewax the slippers or replace them often. Any kind of buildup on the sole can cause a fall. Sometimes a parent does not realize that bread, cake, cookie, or sugar crumbs have been dropped. This residue builds up.

Does your parent have a hearing problem? Determine from the doctor what kind of sound can best be heard with your parent's type of loss. Then have an electrician install the proper buzzer or bell. The telephone company can provide either flashing lights or amplifiers.

Dogs alert people to ringing phones or doorbells. If your parents are fond of pets, they might find that a pet would not only aid them but also be a companion and protector as well.

Should your parent's plight include failing eyesight, magnifying glasses come with a band that fits around the head. Hand-held magnifiers will encompass the entire width of a newspaper column and quite a bit of its length. Magazines and books are now printed in oversized letters. Talking books are available. If your parent enjoys reading the Bible but can no longer do so, not even the large print, there is a complete reading of it on tapes. The reader has a clear, resonant voice, and a blind or nearly blind person can easily keep track of the tape sequence.

Weather also can be a problem. On hot days, encourage your parents to wear loose-fitting, light-colored, lightweight clothing and some kind of ventilated headgear when they go outside. Any yardwork or shopping can be done in the early morning hours.

When winter comes, your parent should never go out without a head covering. More heat dissipates through the top of our heads than from any other part of the body. Layered clothing is warmer. Down-filled stadium jackets and Borgana coats are not only cozy like a fire in a fireplace but lightweight as well. Your parent no longer has to be dragged down by a heavy coat.

Comforters are snug and light. Bed covers no longer need weight to ensure warmth.

In the "Family Doctor" column of *Good Housekeep-*

ing a notation read, "Keep in mind that for elderly people a temperature of 70° F. is none too warm." Help your mother and father understand that a higher electric or gas bill due to keeping the house comfortable is preferable to a case of "accidental" hypothermia which occurs when the core body temperature falls to dangerous levels because the environment is too cool.

An older person also needs safety in other ways. A social security or pension check sent directly to the bank can avert a mugging or the theft of the check.

Being secure within a home is essential for today. A good deadbolt lock on the door and pins in the window frames as well as patio door protection should be installed. Peepholes in the outside doors, if none exist now, should be added. Caution your parent to learn who is asking entrance before opening the door. Also advise your parent that if someone comes to the door wanting to use the telephone because a car has broken down or someone is suddenly ill, the door should remain shut. Your parent, however, can offer to make a call for the person at the door.

Nearly all legitimate service people carry identification cards with their picture. Your loved one should never admit anyone who cannot show such a card. If there is doubt, let the service person wait outside until the company represented has verified the need for the visit. Assure your parent that even if the worker is upset by the delay, it is better to call. Rape, burglary, and vandalism can sometimes be avoided by taking proper precautions.

Remind your parent that answers given to an unknown telephone caller can reveal if a person is alone or widowed. Discuss this. Suggest a reply, such as, "I'd like to check further before answering your questions. Give me the address and telephone number of the company you represent." Then check the telephone directory for its authenticity before calling.

A widow might reply, "I'm sure my husband would not be interested." Remember the old adage, "Forewarned is forearmed." You may save your parent's life or property with these instructions.

On the mailbox or in the telephone directory, be sure to use only initials. If your mother is a widow, she might like your father's initials. Don't use first names for listings, either. This may make an intruder hesitate. It is more difficult to prove the initials are not those of a man.

If your parent lives in a single-family dwelling, think about having floodlights mounted in strategic places. Then any noise or strange sound can be investigated by merely flipping a switch. These lights can be turned on when the house is empty unless the absence of a car would reveal nonoccupancy. There is special equipment that can be installed in a car that will light up a house when you approach. John 3:19 says, ". . . Men loved darkness instead of light, because their deeds were evil."

Do not do what neighbors of ours did while they were away from home. Their son came in every night and turned on some lights. On his way to work each morning, he shut them off. Lights that burn all night are not a safeguard. The day before our neighbors were to return, their home was burglarized. Timers set to turn lights off and on in various parts of the house or to turn the radio on at news time might have prevented their loss.

All these suggestions are important. Do they trigger your own imagination? You know your parents, so you will, no doubt, think of other safety precautions. These can help ensure your parents' survival beyond the Biblical threescore and ten. Be aware. Rectify hazards as you share time and love with your aging parents.

10
Eccentric, Personable, or Mentally Disturbed?

Older people often leave the area of their work when they retire. If this has happened to your parents, you may be astonished at the changes you see in them when you visit.

Does your mother now wear a two-piece bathing suit while swimming off the Gulf Coast of Florida? Has your formerly clean-shaven father grown a beard? Don't be alarmed. Your parents may only be doing what they have wanted to do for years. They may be breaking the bonds that bound them. So be generous in your evaluation of "normalcy." Remember, your parents have a right to live their own lives.

One upsetting difference you may notice as your parents age, however, is the reversal of your roles. One friend told me that as her mother's mental capabilities began to slip, she wanted to be hugged and kissed. When incidents like this begin to happen, it is natural to start to worry, especially if you have counted on your parents for advice and your props are disappearing.

Some aging people demand constant attention. Several friends of mine are provoked whenever the telephone rings. That signal alerts their parents to start asking questions or attempt to get them to hang up. These parents want complete attention and do not wish to share their child.

You can solve this problem. Plan a time for people to call you—a time when your parents are taking a nap or are asleep for the night. Tell your close friends about the arrangement. Offer to call others back at a more convenient time.

Is your parent a worrywart? My mother was. We

lived 500 miles from relatives. Chicago is beautiful but has plenty of crime. I never went on a singing engagement or on a date but what she worried.

Early in my teens I developed a little trick I used all my life. I gave my mother an arrival time of an hour *later* than I anticipated. When I came home on time, she was delighted. I was *early!* I also enjoyed an hour of leeway before I needed to inform her I would be late. When she became confused about the hour I quoted, I wrote it down.

Leaving notes helps, especially if, like a friend's mother, yours latches the storm door and goes to bed and into a deep sleep.

At my suggestion, Alice put a note on the door, "Do not fasten this door." It worked.

Do not simply try to tolerate situations. Search for a solution. You will find it.

Some parents become hypochondriacs, exploit an illness, believe they are persecuted, or use real or imaginary illness to punish their children. The result of this "fakery" may cause us to rebel or act like martyrs. We may accept guilt.

Don't become a martyr. Self-pity is never admirable. It can blight your entire life.

Guilt is an emotion that shackles and wrecks. One doctor says you should never feel guilty if you do what is best for your loved one. He says guilt is a normal response, and every one of us feels it at one time or another. Seeing parents deteriorate can be like watching them die. So the doctor recommends that guilt "be faced, recognized, and worked through in much the same manner."

Guilt may follow our refusal to be dominated. One friend refused to do what her mother dictated. "I will not be bossed," she told her mother, "nor will I explain the reason why I choose to do or not do certain things."

In her case, the mother retaliated by sitting straight

in her chair, her head turned away, her lips tight and pouting. She would not read, watch TV, or speak. The silent treatment and pouting were difficult to endure, especially since the daughter had tried to choose her words carefully and be kind.

When the pressure grew too intense, my friend would sit down at the piano. For her, this became an escape. She discovered it healed her mother's heart, too. Perhaps you can find a common language.

Another daughter with a similar mother chatted away. Normal talk broke down the wall.

I still don't know why my mother would convulse with laughter whenever I used my method. Perhaps because the words I spoke failed to reflect what I did. When she grew angry with me, I would sidle up to her while she was doing the dishes. I'd drape a dishcloth over my arm and say, "Here's your little old Maxine. Always ready *to* help."

"It's hard not to let your parent dominate you," I hear you say. Yes, it is. Especially as you grow older.

A minister mentioned that we must be big individuals when caring for a childish or domineering parent. He maintains we must mature, forsake our own childish ways, and become the controlling factor in our own lives. This minister says the quality that adult children most appreciate in a parent is the lack of bossiness. So try to temper that quality and you'll make life easier.

Other praiseworthy attributes in a parent are compatibility and willingness to carry on household tasks as long as possible.

Stop and think of the good qualities of your parent; then sandwich criticism between two slices of praise. Everyone grows and glows under sincere compliments.

Feeling useful is important. One woman I know lets her mother do the dishes even though she must sometimes rewash them because her mother's eyesight is failing. The daughter makes her mother feel needed.

I recently read about a widower who loved his preschool grandson very much. When the man retired, he dropped in at his daughter's home every day about noon. At first she willingly put another cup and saucer on the table, opened his bakery package, and chatted until Ricky awoke from his nap. They often walked over to the park where the men squatted down to feed the ducks on the pond or squealed in delight at the swings.

Then these visits began to irritate Peggy. While Ricky slept, she wanted to relax.

Peggy's father sensed her irritation even when she didn't say a word. One day he called. "I have a job at the bakery," he said.

Ricky missed his grandpa. So one day Peggy took Ricky to the bakery. The owners didn't even know her father's name. She found him alone, feeding the ducks. They had a good talk, and she let him know he was missed. Then they arranged a compromise.

Now he picks Ricky up and takes him to the park so Peggy has a few hours to herself. He still drops in for lunch at least once a week and they talk. He has become a Mr. Fix-It. Through Peggy, many call him for jobs their husbands either cannot do or do not have the time to accomplish. He is once again useful and active.

Most people enjoy being needed.

Above all, whatever your parent's problem, look for a solution. God promises to provide a way of escape for every testing if you look for it.

Remember, too, that your church, local mental health office, family service association, or city or county office of the aging is there to help you find answers.

Probably one of the hardest crosses to bear is suspicion, another trait of many elderly.

"My children are just waiting for me to die," some parents think, "so they can get my money."

They may be right. A son wheedles the down payment for a house as he thinks, *It will be my money when they die anyway.* If your parent is good enough to lend you money for a down payment, offer to sign a promissory note and make regular payments, plus interest. When you sell the house, be sure to repay the loan immediately.

Most parents worked hard. They scrimped and prayed through depressions and recessions. They saved to give you more than they received. They spent a lifetime arriving at the economic level they now enjoy, so back off on the money issue. Let them do what they want with what is theirs. If you have a catastrophe of a large dimension, of course, your parents may be the first to offer help.

If you back off, it is true your brother or sister may cry "poor mouth" and gain because of it. Communicating may be the key to preventing or rectifying a situation like this.

Once my mother-in-law asked me for some advice about her AT&T rights. When she showed me the two warrants, I noticed the one for the most rights was in her name and that of my husband's brother. After apprising her of the options she had, I told her I knew she wanted to treat her sons fairly and mentioned the unequal division of shares. I suggested she combine them, list all three names, and continue to receive the dividends herself. I never asked her if she followed my advice. When she died, my husband received an equal number of shares. She had done what I suggested.

Your parent's suspicions may center on his or her mate. My friend's father was twenty years older than his wife. When he retired, she continued to work, leaving early in the morning. He was distrustful. He watched her walk to the corner where she caught public transportation. If another man appeared on the street, he interrogated her that night. She repeated in a calm voice that he had no reason to fear.

Keep repeating the truth to a suspicious parent. Perhaps repetition, devoid of anger, will calm this person's spirits. Again, this is the drip-drop method.

It is wise to be aware that suspicion can indicate mental deterioration, such as in the case of my friend's father. Changes in handwriting, dress, cleanliness, and forgetfulness can also be symptoms. (See the appendix for a more complete list.)

Laurence Galton, a medical editor, writer, and visiting professor, says in his book *Don't Give Up on an Aging Parent:* "Senility is *not* invariably linked with hardening of brain arteries. Many symptoms ... can result from emotional reactions to aging, from physical disease ... and from deprivations and insults a long way removed from the brain; ... these are often treatable."

Don't give up on your parents. Don't banish them to an institution. Don't be unkind and say, "They don't know any better" or "Don't pay attention" until you have explored some physical possibilities that may be at the root of their mental problems.

Galton wrote, "The care of the elderly has been largely neglected in the physician's training." The head of a Florida nursing school agrees that nurse's training programs also neglect the care of the elderly.

Don't let this knowledge stop you from exploring what might be wrong with your parent and what can be done. For instance, water on the brain (or hydrocephalus) has long been thought to be a disease of babyhood. Adults, especially the elderly, can develop occult hydrocephalus. A shunt operation, similar to the one done on a child, can reverse some signs of senility. Sophisticated diagnostic techniques are needed for the elderly because many reactions and symptoms in the elderly are different from those of younger people. There can be hope for your parent.

Dicumarol, a blood thinning drug, coupled with psychotherapy is helping some people.

High blood pressure can cause some intellectual decline. Treatment of the pressure can diminish this loss.

Anemia saps the energy of a young person. Your parent may have an iron deficiency anemia that is common in the elderly. A simple blood test will reveal it.

Poor eating habits can be corrected, resulting in an improvement in mental and physical health.

Emphysema, which restricts the amount of oxygen flowing to the brain, can be treated.

Don't rule out thyroid problems. A disorder of this gland can produce mental and emotional disturbances.

Bizarre behavior may be the result of depression brought on by boredom, the deaths of peers, or the fear of death. If you suspect depression, the diagnosis belongs in the hands of an expert.

If your parent complains of muscular pain and weakness and runs a low-grade fever, polymyalgin rheumatica may be the culprit. A blood test revealing a high sedimentation rate and treatment with prednisone can effect a miraculous change.

Don't believe that nothing can be done for your loved one's arthritis. Bed rest, adequate doses of aspirin, and progressive exercises can enable some people to be independent and active, *if the doctor's prescribed treatment is continued.* Cervical osteoarthritis is sometimes helped with hot packs, a cervical collar, and/or surgery. See your parent's doctor or a rheumatologist. Then encourage your parent to continue treatment.

Bad teeth, vitamin deficiency, or drug intoxication can cause mental aberrations. Enlist your parent's doctor in tracking down the culprit.

Remember, too, that memory may decline with age, but in a mentally healthy person, judgment and the ability to appraise a situation *improve* with age.

Some additional facts you should know:

1. Obesity is less ominous in older people.
2. Heart attacks are better at age seventy than at forty.
3. High blood pressure has greater adverse significance in the young.
4. Scientific study indicates that muscle tone and strength can be regained by men who are sixty to ninety years old.
5. Improvement in diet reverses some fatigue, irritability, insomnia, and even confusion. Bone density may be modified.
6. Tooth loss and gum disease are not inevitable.
7. Healthy sexual activity can continue into the eighth and ninth decades.

The ninety-year-old father of a friend announced he planned to marry. His second wife was seventy-eight. He outlived her, maintained mental alertness, and celebrated the 102nd anniversary of his birth.

Juliette K. Arthur has said, "Mental illness is not a disgrace. . . . Approximately one out of every dozen children born each year will sometime . . . suffer a mental illness severe enough to require hospitalization." She advises, "Many who are mentally ill are not hopeless cases."

If your parents become disturbed, *accept them as they have become.* Do not believe they cannot feel anything. Be kind. Speak gently. Pat them on the shoulders or give them a hug. "Love is patient . . . always hopes . . . never fails" (1 Corinthians 13: 4a, 7b, 8a). An unbalanced parent can still feel your love.

Also, find ways to protect your parent as well as yourself. One woman stole into the kitchen at night and turned on the gas jets. Her family protected her by fastening wood panels along the sides of her bed. This protective device allowed her to stay in her familiar surroundings. The panels kept her confined but were no more restraining than the bars of a child's crib.

Margaret W. Wagner, former director of the Benjamin Rose Institute of Cleveland, once said, ". . . unless he is seriously disoriented, destructive, or uncontrollable, the mental institution is not the right place for him."

Some of your strength can be found in the Bible. Read the story of King Jehoshaphat in 2 Chronicles 20. Jehoshaphat was afraid, as many of us are. The enemy was great. But Jehoshaphat knew that "no one can withstand [God]" (verse 6). Do as Jehoshaphat did. Talk to the Lord. Trust Him.

God's Word also tells us a merry heart is like medicine. Keeping your parents happy will provide more mental and physical health for everybody.

Look at the bright things in your life. Shun the drab, depressing ones and love your parents in spite of their idiosyncrasies.

11
Choosing Your Own Way

"Mother, this is the last time," Midge said stepping out the back door. Trudging through the snow, she walked back toward the train. At the store, she avoided the dairy case. She marched toward the prepared cake mixes. This would be a first. She selected brownie packages and chocolate-nut prepared frostings. She reached for paper plates and dropped styrofoam cups into the shopping cart. She also dropped in an advertised brand of instant coffee, a package of teabags, and a box of instant cocoa. Without looking back, she strode straight to the checkout counter.

Later, running water into the sink to wash the silverware, she heard the heavy steps of her mother.

"Margaret Anita Thompson, how—how could you? How *could* you serve packaged mixes on paper plates and instant coffee in paper cups? How could you in my house?"

Slowly Midge turned. "In the future, if you tell me ahead—"

"Tell you ahead of time? I just got the idea at four this afternoon. Besides, the choir was delighted to be invited for your special brownies and whipped cream."

"I'm sure they were, mother, but from now on, such last-minute arrangements will result in prepared mixes and paper plates—or nothing."

Midge held her breath, noticing her mother's cheeks grow pink and her lips purse together. "We'll see," her mother replied as she flounced out of the room.

It isn't easy for most of us to defy a mother. Especially if we're sixty years old, like Midge, and have lived with her all our life. But Midge kept her word.

Lucy had a different problem. When her young niece's husband was killed, Lucy took in her niece's baby, Tim. He lived with Lucy and her mother. Later, Lucy adopted him.

As Tim grew, Lucy's mother seldom agreed with Lucy's decisions about him. Lucy had endured her mother's disagreement in other matters, but Tim was her responsibility. With Tim involved she stood up to her mother.

One time this was extremely hard. Tim ran away. He hated high school. When he returned, he began cutting classes again. One night Lucy said, "If you don't intend to study, you must do something, even if it's joining the Navy."

"Will you sign for me?" he asked eagerly.

"Yes, I'll sign."

That night she took a long walk, her mother's nasty words echoing in her mind. She, too, doubted the wisdom of her decision, but she planned to stand firm. She *would* sign.

In the service, Tim began to value his home, respect Lucy more, and desire an education. After his return, he took a special course and earned his high school diploma. And Lucy had learned to disagree with her mother when she thought it worthwhile.

Sons sometimes have this difficulty with a mother. Vern never dated after he returned from the service. His brothers had married and his sister needed his help for college. His mother made social plans that included both of them. Expecting some relief after his sister's graduation, he was disappointed when she failed to return home. Eventually Vern's mother died. Now he is alone and lonely.

Another man I know has a mother who has cared for his every need and shared most vacations. He has no private life.

If you are the brother or sister of such a man, what

are you doing to ease his burden? Do you take your mother for a weekend or a week so he has time of his own? Do you invite him to go out with you for a time of friendly togetherness, without a parent tagging along? Can you arrange some special vacation for him? Can you care for the parent while he is gone?

Some people bear their own burdens well, but there are times we should heed the Bible's admonition to bear one another's burdens.

If you are the one in such a bind, make a pact with yourself and plan to fill your life with some personal joys. This may mean temporary hurt for your parent. It may prompt some guilt feelings in you. But it can be worth it.

Happiness is not something that comes to us. We make our own. And, like Paul the apostle, we too can find contentment anywhere.

While you are deciding and embarking on a new way, honor your parents. Let them know your love and concern will always be there, even when your way is different from what they would choose for you.

When I hear and see what problems other people have had with their parents, I know I was lucky.

My mother always "campaigned" whenever she knew I had an important decision to make—*until* I weighed all the advantages and disadvantages, asked the Lord about it, and made my final choice. When I told her what I had decided, that was the end of it.

My mother proved different from the mothers of most of my friends; so shortly before her death, I thanked her and asked why she was unusual. She sat a moment, smoothed back her once-auburn hair and lifted her steady gray eyes to gaze into my brown ones. "How could I criticize? I knew you talked decisions over with God. I saw the changes making you happy. Besides, after you'd decided, what was there to say?" I had a great mother.

But you, too, can change things and do what you would like.

I am not an extraordinary person. If I did it, so can you and possibly with more finesse.

It is never too late to say no to your parent.

12
The Death of a Parent

What if one of your parents should die? A death can happen anytime.

If this occurs, please don't pressure your other parent to make decisions immediately. You owe this parent the dignity of making future changes when he or she is not overwhelmed with grief. As in all other circumstances, discover gently and kindly what your parent wishes.

Most people dislike discussing death. It is, however, easier to talk about if your parents are well. Let them tell you, for instance, that they prefer cremation. Even if that is distasteful to you, note their desire and promise to carry it through.

If you live some distance apart, it may be essential to talk about this matter. See if you can convince your mother and father to arrange for a prepaid plan.

Buy your parent a personal record book. These are available at stationery or office supply stores. Sometimes employers offer such booklets. These books have pages to itemize employment benefits, social security numbers, bank and savings and loan accounts, insurance policies (life, household, health, auto, and real estate), U.S. saving bonds, and stocks and bonds. Real estate as well as safe-deposit boxes, wills, cemetery lots, and financial obligations can be shown. Important papers, professional advisors, and other relevant matters can also be listed. Tell your parents that records like these will be valuable to the person who settles the estate.

Many funeral directors are arranging seminars for widows and widowers. Blake-Lamb, a large chain in the

Chicago area, conducts such seminars. They are held once a month (not in the mortuary), and the speakers are bankers, lawyers, and authors like me who have made a new life for themselves. If your parents are separated by death and such seminars are available, urge your living parent to attend. You can go along. If no such meetings are being held, speak to the local funeral director or a community or church leader about starting such sessions.

When Blake-Lamb held their first meeting, they expected about seventy-five widows and widowers. Over 150 came. The refreshments ran out and the sponsors were both surprised and pleased at the response.

When a parent dies, however, let your remaining one adjust to the reality of it. At first there is numbness. It is hard to believe, even if the spouse was seriously or terminally ill.

Of course, some matters must be attended to promptly. Your father or mother should feel strengthened if one of you children accompanies him or her to the bank, the lawyers, the social security office, and any other necessary places.

If you go, don't be nosy. If you are asked for your advice, give choices if you can. Encourage your parent to make the decision. This will initiate independence and avoid repercussions.

Nearly all widows and widowers should stay in their present quarters for six months to a year. This enables them to see whether they can manage alone, whether friends rally round, and whether the place still holds happiness.

These things did not happen with the mother of a friend. My friend visited her mother and talked with her. Because her mother's home was adequate and there was little yard work, my friend and her mother agreed that she could stay on. When this daughter tried to call her mother the next day, however, there was no answer. Finally she called her sister.

"Oh, I bundled mother up and brought her here," said the sister. The mother never returned to her former home.

Try to get the cooperation of your brothers and sisters. Convince them to let your parent be independent. It may not work out, but most people rise to emergencies. Your remaining parent may be stronger than you think.

Sometimes the doctor will tell you it is just a matter of time before your parent will die. Think clearly. The laws of states vary, and if you do not know how yours work, encourage your well parent to withdraw any bank funds.

If you are the joint tenant and your lone parent is dying, withdraw the funds. Keep them intact in another account while you wait to see if some part is to be given to another according to the will. In Illinois, for instance, accounts and safe-deposit boxes are frozen. This could present a problem in paying bills and living expenses.

While your parents are alive, insist they both make a will. A lone parent should also do this. It is the only legal way to indicate his or her wishes.

I can remember doing nothing for my mother when my father died except be at her side at the funeral home and accompany her as she settled things. Yet as I look back, I realize that I gave my mother exactly what she needed. I was there.

I know because my youngest stepdaughter was with us at the hospital as my husband neared the end of his life. Afterward, she followed as her husband-to-be drove me home in my car. Then the Red Cross enabled my Air Force son-in-law, who was in Dayton for a special course, to fly to me rather than return to his base in Madrid, Spain. He was my right-hand man during the first days of my bereavement. I think the nearness of Lorraine and Jack meant more to me than anything else. It may have been the same for my mother.

So be there for your remaining parent. Also remind your father or mother that you are available in the days to come.

Try to keep your brothers and sisters from squabbling. Fighting will not comfort your parent.

Afterward, as has been discussed before, encourage your parent to begin a new life. The longer your mother or father shuts the door and hides any grief, the harder it will be to build fresh happiness.

Let your parent cry. These tears will come unexpectedly and at odd moments, perhaps triggered by the sight of someone's back, the picture of a visited place, the sound of a melody. It is a safety valve—unless it continues too long.

You will notice some things will be easy for your parent. I went to church the day after my husband was buried. I was greeted by a widow who asked, "What are you doing here?"

I replied, "It's Sunday. I belong here." Going to church was easy for me, though I often thought I heard my husband singing behind me in the choir. When I turned to look, he was not there.

Other things may be almost impossible for your parent. Be patient. Show your love. Your father or mother will remember and be grateful.

13
Divorce and Remarriage

In the past most marriages lasted until death. Some withstood the test of time because of love. Others were held together by the inability of a woman to support herself, concern about children, adherence to Biblical teachings, and the stigma of divorce.

Times have changed.

Today more men approaching their middle years struggle with unfulfilled desires and unrest. Because of this, and because less condemnation is attached to divorce, these men are throwing aside marriages of many years.

Women are running away and seeking new experiences at almost epidemic levels. In the future, more freedom for women will probably mean less likelihood they will lean on children for support.

When divorce occurs and both parents are still alive, and if your parents become dependent, where does your allegiance lie? Only you can decide.

Was your father good to your mother? Did your mother treat him fairly? Which one needs you more? Which one do you love best? Is one easier for you to get along with? These are questions to ask yourself. Then, if you cannot care for both and both need help, follow your heart.

But what if your parent, divorced or widowed, wishes to remarry? What will be your reaction? Why will you react that way?

In one episode of "M*A*S*H*" Hawkeye related how he selfishly kept his father from remarrying. He then regretted that his parent was old and without companionship.

The mother of one woman left her daughter's home to marry for the fourth time. The first husband, the daughter's father, had died. The others were shed by divorce. When the mother married the fourth man, the daughter said, "If this marriage doesn't work, I won't take you back." The daughter doubted the new, younger man's sincerity.

When she visited her mother, she often noticed a bruised arm or black eye. The mother always gave a legitimate-sounding excuse. The daughter began to wonder. Was her mother remaining with him because she felt she would have no place to go?

The day a mutual friend asked the younger woman if she knew her stepfather was running around, the daughter went to her mother's home. She found her mother crying. "Does he beat you, too?"

The whispered *yes* was barely audible.

"Pack up your clothes. You're coming home with me."

This mother was an exception, since although men usually remarry, older women seldom do. One of the reasons is the overabundance of available women. Another is that men usually choose younger wives instead of picking one of their peers.

Before the change in the social security law, many older men and women cohabited rather than receive smaller checks due to marriage. Some older people still live together without the strings of a marriage license.

Does this make it the right thing to do? Do you have one set of rules for yourself and another for your remaining parent? Should you encourage remarriage or frown upon it?

One way to answer these questions is to search your own motives. If you oppose a second marriage, are you being selfish or jealous? Are you afraid of losing an inheritance, a baby-sitter, or someone you depend on? Do you know some truth about the proposed spouse that would make him or her unfit for your parent? How do they interact? Do your mother's eyes glow with love? Has your father's energy again become strong?

Love isn't just for the young. An older, companionable marriage, with love, can be the sweetest thing on earth. Age is not even a deterrent to the sexual side.

One woman was widowed for twelve years before she found the right partner. The husband-to-be was unexpectedly hospitalized but released before the wedding date, though test results were not yet available. They married. When the test results showed cancer, he said, "I would never have married you."

"I would have insisted anyway," his bride replied. "You'll be fine."

Her two married daughters wondered what the future held for their mother. They worried about her. The husband did not recover from his cancer; he lived just over a year. His wife nursed him as well as if they had been married many years. She made his last days peaceful.

In view of the prospective results of the tests, should the wedding have been postponed? Should the plans have been canceled?

It's hard to say. Some children would have insisted that their mother wait. But what would have been accomplished? The results would probably have forced him to call off the wedding. The mother would have had a difficult decision. Agreeing to stop the wedding would have hurt him even if it was the right thing to do. If they had married, would he have believed she married him out of pity?

Second marriages are quite common. The ones I know about don't seem to be having trouble with their children, and the offspring are not burdened, even though many of the couples are in their seventies and eighties.

Perhaps love and friendship in later years keep health and spirits strong. Eating with a companion is more enjoyable than eating alone; the warmth of another body is better than the pristine coolness of sheets.

Nevertheless, you are right to try to ensure that this prospective marriage will be a good one. To do so, consider the following questions:

Has the future bride or groom been widowed or divorced? How many times?

What kind of temperament does each person have? Do they appear compatible?

If there are children from previous marriages, if there had been a divorce, if the divorce was effected in a different state, if community property is involved, or if one of them is financially better off, a premarital agreement might be wise. An agreement like this is no longer just for the rich.

You may want to find out what kind of financial arrangement has been made in case of the death of either spouse. In one marriage the widow sold her house and moved to the man's. He died four years later. He left her a lifetime interest in his house, which was to go to the church when she died. He thought he was providing for her. Within a few years, however, she could not take care of it. She wound up living with a stepdaughter from her first marriage.

One thing you should insist upon is a will.

I had never been married when I accepted the proposal of my husband who was at that time a widower. When he said he was going to make out a new will, I said, "I must have one, too." He disagreed.

I explained that if we were both killed in an accident and I outlived him by one minute, his girls could be cut off without a cent. The relatives I hadn't seen in years could file a claim.

"Max is right," the lawyer said.

So insist your parent and his or her prospective spouse each draw up a will.

If one person dies, have arrangements been made for the care of the stepfather or stepmother? Will they become your responsibility? Find out.

What is planned for the furniture and belongings when the two households are joined? Maybe you are worried about treasures. Is there something your parent has that you have loved? If this parent plans to remarry, ask him or her if you can either have it now or if it can be put into the will for you.

It is sad when an in-law or sibling strips a residence of diamond rings, a precious gift you gave a parent, or some other item. Try to prevent this from happening if you can. Asking ahead of time is one way.

Once you agree that marriage is right for your parent, sit back and watch him or her glow.

Sometimes there is cause to protest. If your father picks up someone off the street, speak to him lovingly. Ask his minister, priest, or lawyer to discuss it. Request a couple who loves your father to talk with him. Pray about it.

One daughter disliked the man her mother dated and made comments like: "His nose is so big." "He's so much older." "He'll be an invalid and you'll be stuck." "Did you notice his dirty fingernails?" "How can you stand the way he eats?" Those who knew this daughter felt sure she was jealous. Her mother could get a suitor while she could not.

Just as many women can see the subterfuge in another woman, so men can spot falseness in those of their sex. One young man became suspicious of the handsome, rugged person who was escorting his mother. This son wanted happiness for his mother but doubted she would find it with this man. He didn't want to tell his mother his suspicions; he chose, instead, to gather facts to present to his mother. The son discovered that the man who was dating his mother was a fraud, a con man. The son exposed him to his mother just before the FBI made the arrest.

Opposition can be wise. If you dislike a woman who is flirting with your father or if you mistrust a man who is dating your mother, sift your motives and base your opposition on facts.

Love is different the second time around. Many times it is serene rather than exciting, calm instead of fevered, deep rather than surface infatuation. This does not mean it is any less powerful or lasting. Love is not just for the young. Fire can be kindled in older hearts, and love can shine from fading eyes.

If you do not agree with some of the arrangements of the prospective marriage, organize your complaints along with some suggestions and present these to your parent in a calm, sincere voice. There may be merit in your thinking; your parent may realize this and make adjustments.

Whatever you do, however, do not fall into the trap of believing your parent is too old for "this sort of stuff." One is never too old for love. Support your parent in every way you can and give him or her your blessing.

14
What About Your Own Romance?

"You're going to be a missionary?" I overheard my mother say to a young man. "Well, my daughter can't stand bugs and snakes."

At another time she laughed and remarked to a lad, "I've never been able to interest Maxine in cooking."

But I became angry enough to say so when my mother told one boyfriend, "If you can't pick up my daughter at her door, just forget about going out with her." My mother knew he worked at a radio station with extended programming in summer and that he always arranged for my dinner while I waited for him. His school was strict with a curfew. He always brought me home. This meant he had to sign a late sheet.

The boys I liked, she didn't; the ones I couldn't stand, she pushed. Was this her "game"—trying, consciously or unconsciously, to keep me with her? When I confronted her, she denied trying to discourage these young men. After that, however, we did not have another problem.

Just as I had arguments with my parent regarding dates, so may you. I believe these parental actions are not always a *conscious* attempt to keep you with them. But parents can use various ploys.

One day my husband and I visited my best friend, Louise, and her mother. The mother lay in a bed in the living room facing the TV. During our entire visit, the mother neither moved nor looked at us.

"What does the doctor say, Lou?" I asked later.

"He says there's something bothering her and nothing physically is wrong. I don't understand it."

Later on the doctor questioned Lou. "There has to be something upsetting your mother," he said. "Think!"

Louise pondered a moment. "Well, she doesn't like my boyfriend."

"That's it," the doctor exclaimed. "She doesn't want to lose you."

Lou hated to believe it, but when she broke up with Nick, her mother made a miraculous recovery.

Mary became engaged to a man about twelve years her senior. They rented an apartment and she prepared it for the wedding day.

"Mother's not well," he said. "I can't leave her." This kind of postponement continued for fifteen years.

Five years into the relationship I had told her, "He'll never marry you. When a man really wants a wife, he finds a way. If you wait around, he'll pick someone younger, and you will have wasted the best years of your life."

That is exactly what happened.

Enid and Dave went together for twenty years. Both supported dependent mothers, so both love and empathy bound them together. One day a widower asked Enid for a date. In less than six months, Enid and the widower were engaged.

"I can't believe it," Dave said. "We had an understanding. How can she love someone else?" He was crushed. He was also blind. When her evenings became too busy, shouldn't he have guessed the reason? She was attractive. If he really loved her, don't you think he could have made more of an effort to keep her?

Have you ever walked in Enid's, Dave's, or Mary's shoes? Did you feel trapped? Has parental responsibility kept you from marriage?

Ann Landers once wrote, "Enjoy yourself. A woman of forty should not have to live her life to please her mother."

One minister said, "Don't let parents dictate the relationship. Don't allow the parent to control ... through little 'games'. . . ."

Romance for single and married children can be inhibited or nonexistent when we care for dependent parents. Can we solve this problem? We can try.

Once I told Lola, whose mother was trying to break up her attachment for a man, "I think your mother's afraid for herself. Life with one of your siblings would not be smooth. Either make a break with the fellow and stick to your guns or tell your mother you're going to marry this man."

Several months later Lola spoke to her sisters and brothers. "I'm marrying, but I want one year to adjust without ma. I'll take her back, but I'd like you to share her now."

Lola's siblings agreed. She and Niles married. Everything proceeded smoothly except for the mother's resentment. "You're putting me out in the street," she complained.

The newlyweds were happy until it was Lola's little brother's turn. He was the father of several children, over forty, his mother's favorite, and the baby in the family. At two o'clock one morning he telephoned Lola. "Come and get *your* mother," he said. Lola did.

Later I rejoiced when the mother told me, "Niles is good to Lola. Both are kind to me."

The mother of another friend of mine deliberately broke up a serious romance. "I'll never again let her know when I'm getting married until the last day," my friend said. And she almost succeeded. Due to her future husband's prospective transfer, however, the news had to be made known in advance.

"My life has been hell since she's known," she told me.

At the wedding, when the minister asked for objections, my husband saw a brother cover the mother's mouth. At the reception, the mother wept and wailed. Now the mother believes he is the best of her sons-in-law.

God can lead you out of any maze. You who do not believe in God can do the same thing as a believer. Push aside your emotional instincts. Think logically and realistically about your problem. Solve it.

Sometimes discussing your dilemma with a friend will trigger a solution. It may be a solution your heart does not want to accept, but it may unveil your "way of escape."

Mary, the woman engaged to the older man, was not as fortunate as the others I have mentioned. When her man married another woman, Mary's youth was gone, the best men were married, and her own mother was partially dependent upon her.

Act before this happens to you. But try to empathize with your parent. He or she may possess wounds you will never know about. You can accept the thorns in your life and grow roses in spite of them.

Don't let the years keep passing you by. If marriage is your dream, it can come true. Go to night school or to new activities, alone. Yes, *alone.* Some men are scared off if a woman always has a female friend in tow.

One friend of mine loved piano music and was herself an accomplished pianist. She liked a special section of seats in Chicago's Orchestra Hall and bought two season tickets to the Sunday afternoon concerts so she could invite a friend. One year, short of cash because her mother had undergone a costly operation, she cut expenses by buying only one ticket for the season.

In the lobby one Sunday, a young man started to talk with her. The next Sunday he invited her to dinner after the performance. They discussed the concert and music in general. He drove her home and asked for a real date. Later, he admitted he had been watching her, but she was always with a friend. "I didn't want to butt in," he said.

No marriage developed from their friendship, but it could have. She learned the lesson that being alone does not necessarily mean you will stay that way.

Widen your horizon. Nothing says you must sit at home knitting at your mother's knee, caring for the cats, and hoping the telephone will ring.

One woman loved to eat and her mother loved to cook. As the woman enjoyed her mother's abundant cooking, she also gained weight. She took the position that she was not going to spoil her mother's loving efforts by refusing to eat in the hopes someone would fall in love with her. Her personality and dress would have to speak for her.

One day she was seated between two attractive men on a transcontinental flight. She thought, *I'm not going to allow these men to believe I'm just a tall, fat hulk.* She began talking. They discussed many subjects.

One of them, a dress designer, was planning a new line for heavier women. He needed a personable ambassador to travel and display his designs. Just prior to their arrival at their destination, the dress designer handed her his card. "If you are ever interested in a new job," he said, "please contact me."

"I'm going," she told her mother. And now she is married to a very fine person who loves her for what she is.

When you are married, you may experience different problems. One of my friends is a Christian saint. When her husband's father was operated on and given six months to live, she said, "Let's take him in. We'll sleep in the basement since my mother occupies the other bedroom. The basement will give us some privacy."

It has been five years since the father arrived. He

wears a permanent catheter and often has an accident just before company is to arrive. His son is given four weeks vacation with pay each year, but the time is spent at the house.

Once, when the couple wanted to take an out-of-town trip, a brother said, "Can't your wife's mother take care of pa?" This little mother does mighty well to take care of most of her own needs.

Finally this couple did get away for a short time, but the wife had to speak up for it to happen.

Speaking up and privacy are both needed to keep a marriage vibrant when a parent lives with you.

And with a live-in parent, some people become inhibited about love-making—perhaps dating back to childhood and a parent's admonitions about purity. There is a solution to this, too.

Run away. Spend a weekend in an expensive motel. Have a wonderful second honeymoon.

One couple who shared their home with their parents and did not have much money had a younger sister who always surfaced with a problem every time the couple talked about starting a family. Luke and Mildred decided to be selfish. Within a few years they became the parents of two lovely girls. Mildred's parents got the joy of "spoiling" grandchildren. Sis learned to stand on her own feet.

A decision that seems to benefit you alone may also bring joy and maturity to others. My husband made such a decision.

When his first wife died, his mother-in-law lived in their home. She tried to stop him from changing the interior, giving mementos to his wife's close friends; she also discouraged dating. Finally he told his sister-in-law who lived nearby, "I have my own mother to consider. Your mother belongs with her own children." He needed a chance to rebuild his life and to fall in love again. He did not feel guilty about this. Nor should you.

A minister said, "We must not feel guilty about putting our immediate family first. The parent problem may have no solution."

God's Word says a man and woman should *leave* father and mother and cleave to the spouse. We should stand united.

Speaking out may solve our problems, but speak in love.

If you ask God for understanding and analyze the circumstances, you should find a way to keep romance in your life.

15
Your Dreams, Your Goals, and God's Promises

Hold fast to your dreams for a lost dream is like a bird with a broken wing trying to fly.

(Wall of the Dallas airport)

I slid onto the stool in the tiny restaurant and looked up at the waitress. Right then I knew I should not let astonishment show in my eyes. But it already had.

A little later, as Jean set down a cup of coffee in front of me, she said, "Wait until nine and you can have company home." Something about the way she said it made me think it was she who wanted the company.

When we last met, she had been working as a legal secretary. *What was she doing now behind the counter of a two-bit restaurant?* Somewhere deep inside of me rose a possible clue. Was she doing what I wanted, too? Was she overturning her restricted world and walking in the light of her fire?

I hadn't long to wait for answers.

Her laughter rang out as we pulled up our coat collars against the chill wind and hurried up the steps to the elevated train station. "Guess you wonder what I'm doing behind a lunch counter," she said as we sank down on the "three-for-a-nickel" seat in the coach. She plopped an armload of books between us and settled back into the corner. Before I could reply, she continued, "I'm doing the most insane, idiotic thing of my whole life."

"It's agreeing with you!"

"It is. But most of my friends think I've gone bananas."

Then she told me the story. Jean had made up her mind when she was thirty-eight that she would enter teacher's college if she could pass the entrance exams. Figuring out her expenses, she discovered scrimping would make it financially possible. Her father's bout with cancer seemed to be victorious. The need to supplement the family income no longer existed.

"I decided I must do it," she told me, "while there is still time."

"You've always adored children," I said. "A secretarial job should be easy to find if this doesn't work."

"Then you're about the only one who agrees. But, I'm determined. I feel God is leading me."

Every speck of Jean's determination and faith was required when the cancer returned, this time to her father's throat. As he lay dying in the rented hospital bed, she relieved her mother at night. She pushed herself. She cut her school load, extended her work hours. Her dream still lived.

Standing at her mother's right beside her father's casket, the fine, high cheekbones above lean cheeks made her dark-circled eyes look even larger. She steadied her out-of-date pillbox hat self-consciously from time to time, but her eyes were luminous, her smile sweet. She had succeeded in discharging her responsibility with honor and had kept faith in her dream.

We now live many miles apart and Jean has never married. But God has set her in a family as He promised in Psalm 68:6, a family so heterogeneous it is a constant challenge and joy.

It can be the same for you.

Vi, the friend who pinned the note on my calendar pad that January day, had a different kind of dream. She longed to serve God as a Poor Clare nun. Just when she thought her dream was materializing, her mother suffered a heart attack. Her parents needed her at home.

She spent two years rushing her mother to the hospital for each successive attack. After her mother's death, she returned to her former job.

We carried on many religious discussions. One tenet she held was that the greatest gift we can give to God is to sacrifice our desires and talents for His service.

Vi did not know if the order would accept her. She was now over thirty, the maximum age for admittance.

When I could not convince her that God does not want sacrifice, I realized I had no right to try to change her thinking if God had pointed her in a certain direction. I then offered to pray for her to be accepted into the order. God answered our prayers.

The day she left for the convent we laughed together as we admired the sparkling ring on my third finger, left hand. Marriage had not been my dream. In my fantasies I sang from the stage of Chicago's Orchestra Hall; I saw strange oceans and mountains and picturesque countries; I picked up magazines and books and saw my name on them. These dreams, all of them, began when I was eight or nine, when off-key songs began filling our flat, when I riffled through my geography book, when I sold my first poem.

When I was thirteen, God turned my heart to Himself and tuned my out-of-pitch vocal chords. I was on my way to my second dream.

Every year of my early childhood we journeyed to my grandparents' home in the heart of Missouri. My father was a railroad worker who was allowed two "foreign" passes a year. I begged to go to other places—just once.

My dream of traveling is now being realized, too. I have been all over the United States and Canada, to Europe, the British Isles, Australia, New Zealand, even to Tahiti.

I expect writing to be the last of my complete

fulfillments, though it was the first success on my wishing road.

What are the essential ingredients for making a dream walk? First, I believe, is confidence. God-confidence and self-confidence. Have faith. Believe.

Of course, you need a little more than faith. You need stick-to-it-iveness.

Most of us find time to do the things we really want to do, only sometimes it is like conquering a barbed-wire fence. On my grandparents' farm I learned how to get through such fences. You separate the wires and fling your leg through again and again. You get scratched on the way, but trouble is a part of life.

It's up to you. How much struggling will you endure for the realization of your dream? How long can you wait?

One thing is sure. Nothing will thrill you so much as succeeding at something you thought was unattainable. To reach it while obeying the only commandment of God that holds a promise is doubling your accomplishment.

That commandment says:

Honor your father and your mother, so that you may live long in the land the Lord your God is giving you (Exodus 20:12).

Honor. It's a word that does not seem to mean much in today's political arena or even in some personal relations.

In the commandment it is an action verb. *Roget's Thesaurus* says to honor is to "do one's duty, discharge one's function, stay at one's post, go down with one's ship, come up to what is expected of one, not to be found wanting, keep faith with one's conscience, face one's obligations, redeem a pledge" and "pay up," among other definitions. To honor someone is a big order.

Most of us do not fulfill this in its entirety. When this fact jars our conscience, we feel guilty. But guilt is not the proper emotion if our deeds are the best we can do. God does not expect perfection. Only Jesus, the God-Man, is perfect. If we were also perfect, what would be the reason for His coming, and how could we know the peace of His forgiveness?

The commandment about our duty to our parents is the only one of ten to include a promise.

Neither I nor many of the friends I mentioned in this book have lived long enough for me to say that long life is given when you honor and care for parents. But if we assume that part of the promise includes the giving of land, and if we can prove those who kept the commandment received it, isn't it logical to assume that the rest of the promise will be kept?

To check this, I reviewed the previous pages of this book and made a list. Of the people I have mentioned, I have lost track of four. The Poor Clare nun has taken a vow of poverty. One man and one woman do not hold a deed to property.

However, *more than 75 percent of all the rest* became property owners *after* the death of their parents. This assures me that God keeps His whole promise.

I am one of the 75 percent. Had anyone told me I would gain property after caring for my parents, I would have laughed. Some might say I am an owner only because my husband died and I inherited it. I believe that is but half the story.

When I shouldered the burden of caring for my parents, I did it because they had no other child. Perhaps that is why I never became bitter or felt trapped. Many people, however, would call it my cross.

Only a couple of years ago a minister talked about the crosses we are called upon to bear. Now, I am no Pollyanna, but I couldn't think of a single cross I've borne. I believe ⁀his is the "fault" of my wonderful Lord.

If caring for my parents was my cross—my yoke—
it was easy and the burden was light. It can be light for
you, too.

Recently I was rereading Jeremiah and came upon
a portion I had never noticed before. In Jeremiah 23:33
the words that stood out for me were these: "When this
people . . . ask thee, saying, what is the burden of the
Lord? thou shalt . . . say . . . what burden?" (KJV). Truly
the care of our parents need not be a burden.

Love them, communicate with them, care for them
to the best of your ability, and when they have left you,
look forward to the promise of God. Remember that
one of His promises is of a place not made with hands,
eternal in the heavens, and prepared for us.

Is heaven the "land" in the commandment? I don't
know. I am only sure that I serve a wonderful Father.

I cannot lose, either here or hereafter!

APPENDIX

PROTECTIVE SERVICES ACT 166

This act:

1. Prohibits abuse or the allowing of abuse of developmentally disabled adults and persons suffering infirmities of aging or other like incapacities.

2. Requires reporting of incidents of adult abuse to the Office on Aging.

3. Establishes a Central Registry of reported instances of adult abuse and

4. Provides for the possibility of protective services (even temporary or long-term protective custody) for those individuals unable to protect themselves.

This includes any willful or negligent acts that result in neglect, malnutrition, sexual abuse, unreasonable physical injury, endangerment to mental health, unjust or improper use of an adult for one's own advantage, and failure to provide necessary treatment, attention, sustenance, clothing, shelter, or medical services.

If you wish to report such abuse, you will need the following information:

1. Name, address, and telephone number of the person allegedly abused, neglected, or exploited.

2. Age, sex, and race.

3. Description of the problem.

4. Name and address of person inflicting abuse, neglect, or exploitation.

5. Relationship of the abuser to the victim.

6. Name and address of the person reporting.

In Arkansas, reports are to be made to the Arkansas Office on Aging, Advocacy Assistant Program, Donaghey Building, Suite 1428, Little Rock, Arkansas, 72201. Or a free call can be made from anywhere in Arkansas to 1-800-482-8049.

CHOOSING A HOME
QUESTIONS COMPILED BY THE ILLINOIS
COUNCIL FOR LONG-TERM CARE

Questions to Ask:

1. Is the home licensed? Ask. If the answer is yes, ask to see the license. Government experts advise that if a home is not licensed, you should not even consider it.

2. Does the administrator have a current state license? Again, if the answer is yes, ask to see it.

3. Is the nursing home approved by Medicare and Medicaid?

4. What other insurance plans are accepted?

5. Are there additional charges for personal laundry? Does therapy cost extra? If so, how much? Obtain a written list of services included, as well as a list of services furnished at extra cost. Check how often rates have been raised.

6. Are residents allowed to furnish their own rooms with their own furniture? Can residents use their own radio or television? Are the rooms clean, pleasant, and comfortable? Does the place smell of urine or any other unpleasant odor?

7. Can a husband and wife share the same room?

8. Can residents have alcohol? Can they smoke in their room unsupervised? Are there other convenient places where smoking is permitted?

9. Are there restrictions on making and receiving phone calls? Is a telephone readily available or can one be connected in the patient's room?

10. What are the visiting hours? Is the resident allowed to visit friends and relatives outside the nursing home? If visiting hours are restricted, be suspicious of the place.

11. Where is the resident's money kept? Are there provisions for personal banking services? Are accurate records kept of residents' financial transactions?

12. Does each resident have his or her own closet and chest of drawers?

13. What is the capacity of the home? How many residents are presently there? How many people share a room?

14. Are the residents encouraged to leave their rooms when able? What are the grounds like? Is the place located so patients can safely go for walks? Walking is the best exercise. (One nursing home in my area faces a busy state road. If the occupants of the home walk, they must do it on the shoulders of the road. Regulations governing nursing, board-and-care homes, and other types differ. In some states a nursing home is forbidden to locate on such sites, while a board-and-care home may do so.)

15. When was the last state or local inspection? You may want to see the most recent inspection report.

16. How often are fire drills held for the staff and residents? Are federal and/or state fire codes met? Is there a written emergency evacuation plan? Are emergency exits marked? Are there grips and railings in the bathrooms and hallways? If the building is two to five stories high, is there a way to get the patients out in case of a fire?

17. What types of activities are available to residents? Don't hesitate to ask to see the schedule of activities. Try to speak with patients or their relatives and ask for their views. Ask about the staff turnover. It is high in many homes, sometimes with good reason. It is difficult to watch people deteriorate, and working with older people can become depressing.

18. How are the residents' medical needs met? Does the nursing home have an arrangement with a nearby hospital to handle emergencies? Is a physician available at all times? Can the patient use his or her own doctor? Is a registered nurse in charge at all times? What is the patient-staff ratio? Is it adequate? (H. Terri Brower, a professor of nursing at the University of Miami's School of Nursing, says, "Nurses who work in nursing homes traditionally have been stigmatized by their professional peers." She also says nursing schools are not doing enough to prepare their graduates to work with the elderly and that there is no special training in gerontology.)

19. Is there a dining hall or do residents eat in their rooms? Are special diets available for those who need them?

If not, is there a professional dietician on the staff, available as a consultant? Is food well-prepared and nutritious? Are kitchen and dining areas sanitary? Are patients helped to eat? Is adequate time allowed for meals? Are snacks available? (Try to visit the home during a mealtime. Talk to some of the residents. Get their opinions of the meals.)

Juliette K. Arthur in her book *How to Help Older People* says, "Mental illness gives warning. . . . Recognize . . . that a man or woman may need psychiatric care if he:

1. lives in a separate world and fails to face his problems;

2. has severe 'blues' to such an extent that he is unable to carry on his everyday activities;

3. suffers agonies of indecision . . . then obstinately refuses to carry out some plan even if it is to his advantage;

4. has a delusion that you or someone else is persecuting him;

5. has moods which swing like the pendulum . . . ;

6. insists he is ill, complains continually of aches and pains, and a variety of bodily deviations which a thorough physical examination reveals nothing. . . . [This sixth point may be misunderstood. Once my husband went to five doctors seeking medical help. All stated, "Nothing wrong." On the last occasion I went with him. Because I knew my husband, I convinced the doctor to check further. This doctor found the cause. Know your parent. He or she may be ill.]

7. cannot sleep without medication, or relapses into apathy and listlessness;

8. is excessively irritable and given to outbursts of rage;

9. loses interest in his appearance, his environment, and his family;

10. talks feverishly and constantly, repeating the same things . . . ;

11. goes on spending sprees . . . hoards every cent—his clothes, his food—without reason;

12. is a prey to unfounded anxieties about everything;

13. sees or hears imaginary things and people."

INDEX

Health: eating habits, 28, 76, 88, 89, 102; general, 18, 27, 42, 51; home care, 55; medical care, 18, 19, 56, 57, 75, 76, 79, 97; medications, 58, 76, 87; mental, 56, 57, 58, 82, 83, 85–90 *passim*, 105, 106, Appendix 119; safety, 47; stroke, 53, 60; your own, 39.

Home ownership: disadvantages of, 19, 32, 115–117 *passim*.

Honor: 115, 116.

Hospices: 55.

Independence: encouragement of, 38, 39; loss of, 24, 25; submission to, 25.

Individuality: 10, 22, 23, 32.

Laws: regarding abuse of a parent, 54, 100, Appendix 118; regarding support of a parent, 37, 38.

Legal services: *See* Protective Services, 54.

Listening: to your parents, 16, 15, 66.

Living arrangements: independent, 32, 66, 96; joining generations, 35, 36, 39–44, 46, 47, 55; nursing homes, 53, 56–61, 65, 69, 70; nursing homes, choice of, Appendix 119–121; *passim*; nursing homes improvements of, 64; nursing homes types, 63; when is care necessary, 56, 58, 60, 61; with another, 32, 33, 39, 63.

Love: 10, 52.

Marriage: general, 46; your own, 46, 50, 53, 56, 67, 68, 109–111, 114.

Moving: considerations of, 19, 20, 25, 26, 32, 48, 82.

Nursing homes: *See* Living arrangement.

Nutrition: inside home, 27–31, 88; outside of home, 28.

Office on Aging: *See* Protective Services.

Ombudsman/Advocate Program: 60, 62, 63.

Organizations for the elderly: *See* Agencies.

Patients' rights: 64.

Peace: of mind, 10, 11, 35, 36, 59, 116.

Prayer: how to and when, 15, 31, 56, 58, 59, 66, 90, 93, 103, 111, 115.

Preplanning for parents' old age: drip-drop method, 16, 87; family leader, 44, 45; financial, 50; general, 12, 46, 48, 49; how to talk about it, 16, 64, 65; living quarters, 12, 17, 31, 55, 57, 60; suggestions, 16, 46, 60.

Problems: abuse, (*See* Protective Services, 54); adult grandchildren, 42, 49; children, 49, 50, 92, 102; controversy, 41, 91, 92; driving ability, 17, 75, 76; employment of son or daughter, 13; entertainment, 43; personality clashes, 44, 47, 48, 49; physical, 17–19, 56, 57, 75, 76; prevention of, 21, 22, 32, 33, 36, 37, 44, 47, 48, 49; privacy, 43, 51, 52, 109, 110; similarity, 10, 42, 47; temperature, 79, 80; time use, 27, 62; vacations, 44, 51, 109, 110.

Protective Services: 53, 54, 60, 61, Appendix 118.